The Drama Therapy Decision Tree

The Drama Therapy Decision Tree

Connecting Drama Therapy Interventions to Treatment

Paige Dickinson and Sally Bailey

intellect

Bristol, UK / Chicago, USA

First published in the UK in 2021 by
Intellect, The Mill, Parnall Road, Fishponds, Bristol, BS16 3JG, UK

First published in the USA in 2021 by
Intellect, The University of Chicago Press, 1427 E. 60th Street,
Chicago, IL 60637, USA

A catalogue record for this book is available from
the British Library.

Copy editor: Newgen KnowledgeWorks
Cover designer: Aleksandra Szumlas
Production manager: Aimée Bates
Typesetting: Newgen KnowledgeWorks

Print ISBN 978-1-78938-247-1
ePDF ISBN 978-1-78938-248-8
ePub ISBN 978-1-78938-249-5

This is a peer-reviewed publication.

Contents

Acknowledgments vii
Prologue ix

SECTION 1: FOUNDATIONS 1

1. Foundational Principles of the Therapeutic Process 3
2. Foundational Principles of Drama Therapy 21
3. Foundations of Diagnoses and Global Functioning 39

SECTION 2: THE DRAMA THERAPY DECISION TREE 73

4. A Systematic Method of Drama Therapy Treatment Planning 75
5. A Systematic Method for Choosing Drama Therapy Interventions 95
6. A Systematic Method for Drama Therapy Treatment Evaluation 123

SECTION 3: DIVERSITY AND ETHICAL CONSIDERATIONS 143

7. Diversity: Cultural Competence, Adaptations and Accommodations 145
8. Ethics 175

Appendix A The Drama Therapy Decision Tree 203
Appendix B Global Outcomes Connected to Drama Therapy Intervention Suggestions 225
References 245
Index 257

Acknowledgments

We would like to thank the people who have supported us during the writing of this book.

We were inspired to write this book by our students at Kansas State University and Eckerd College, who kept asking for a resource detailing how to synthesize all the information we were pouring into their brains. Right before we started writing, Sally's supervision class practiced brainstorming which drama therapy interventions would work with specific DSM diagnoses and why. They said they wanted credit when the book came out, so here it is: Michael Rogers, Sarah Edwards, Funmilola Cole, Sherry Brown, Soekie Woolls, Hannah Rockey, Ellen Burke, and Tim Tarkelly.

To the editors at Intellect who responded within eight weeks to our query and accepted our book proposal. They have been accessible and helpful whenever we needed them: Amy Damutz, Tim Mitchell, Jessica Lovett, Naomi Curston, and Aimee Bates. APA format is ingrained in our brains. We are so grateful that the Intellect team was willing to work in APA format, so our brains did not have to do contortions to remember a different citation style!

In terms of artwork, we could not be more pleased with the cover design created by Alex Szumlas. We do a "happy dance" each time we look at it. Thanks also to Sue Leo for her infographic of the Drama Therapy Pie and Hunter Pressley for her wonderful depiction of the Drama Therapy Decision Tree in the Prologue.

Thanks to the colleagues who read various sections of the manuscript and served as experts on special populations or adaptations/accommodations: Nicole Andrusky-Harris and Kristin Long for their knowledge of Deaf culture and cochlear implants, Hunter Blencowe and Ally Gallagher for their expertise in animal assisted therapy and service animals, and Susana Pendzik for feedback on all we wrote about her construct of dramatic reality and the six keys. Thanks to Lanell Finneran for brainstorming book titles, reading several early chapters, and for providing laughs and an introduction to Ninja Ginger Chips. Thanks also to Calli Armstrong for surveying the drama therapy community to confirm which diagnoses drama therapists most frequently address so that our case studies would be most relevant to readers. We are exceedingly grateful to Dr. Mimi Savage for her careful and cogent suggestions about the text and her support and enthusiasm for it. We know she was very busy at the time, and we appreciate her giving of her time and energy to our work.

We were sustained in our work by the enthusiasm of the many drama therapists who attended our workshops at the North American Drama Therapy Conferences during the beginning stages of the Drama Therapy Decision Tree. Whenever we have emailed them for suggestions, they have responded to our queries and encouraged us (as in "So WHEN is the book coming out?")

Most importantly, thanks go to Quincy, Fred, and Tucker, our cats, who provided comic relief and lots of unconditional positive regard throughout long hours of writing together in-person and on the phone.

Prologue

Entering the profession of drama therapy, the authors of this book walked in to lead our first drama therapy groups knowing that just playing theatre games or improvising scenes was not enough, yet we felt at a loss as to how to proceed in a systematic and effective therapeutic manner. We had been trained in a variety of drama therapy interventions and methods (e.g., role method, psychodrama, sociodrama, playback theatre, etc.), we had taken courses in abnormal psychology, group processes, theories of counseling, and life span development. We could watch a drama therapist in action and identify what theory was being used, why the theory did or did not work, and we could rattle off the interventions that were being employed. But we had difficulty reversing that process. We had difficulty looking at a new group and saying, "This is what is dysfunctional in these clients, and this is how I can use drama therapy to intervene." We wondered how the drama therapists, who were our mentors and supervisors, knew what to do for which participants at different times. In short, we felt overwhelmed.

Even though we had been taught systematically, our knowledge was not cohesive; it was more like disconnected pieces of a thousand-piece puzzle. We had the puzzle pieces, but we did not know how to start putting them together to create a complete picture. People who do puzzles all the time have a system. They will tell you:

> First pull out the edge pieces, then start sorting colors together, and then work on the puzzle in sections. Take the edge pieces and build the frame of the puzzle, then put together the distinct imagery, and then the background. The sections get bigger and start fitting together with each other. Voilà, the puzzle is complete.

We needed a system like that.

Part of the struggle that most early career professionals face relates to the way much of higher education is delivered. All the pieces of information are presented separately in different semesters and not always presented in relation to each other. That is not done to confuse students; the reality is that only one piece of information can be learned at a time. Additionally, when one skill builds upon another, the first must be taught before the next. For instance, a student cannot learn how an intervention will affect a population (i.e., a group of people with a specific diagnosis) without learning first about the intervention and then about the population. Drama therapy students might learn the empty chair technique in a psychodrama class in the fall, but not in context with a specific population. Abnormal psychology, which provides information about specific diagnostic populations, might be taught in a different semester. Drama therapy with special populations provides instruction on how to adapt the empty chair for a particular population, and that course might be in yet another semester. Realistically, there is not enough time in a two- to three-year master's degree program to explore all the combinations of diagnoses and interventions that might be needed in practice. Even in a doctoral program there is no way to take enough classes to understand all the combinations of participants, interventions, and practice situations that exist in the real world.

What each of us separately discovered, as we grew as therapists and teachers, was a way to synthesize our separate areas of knowledge into a body of knowledge that was accessible to us when needed. Rather than floundering around for ten years, we would like every drama therapist to be able to start thinking systematically right at the beginning of their career. We hope this book will provide that system for you.

This book presents the drama therapy decision tree, which integrates the components involved in drama therapy practice. Using the decision tree as a guide, early career drama therapists can move forward confidently and ground their work with participants in an integrated system. This does not mean that you will never feel confused or that you will never make a mistake, but we hope that you will feel more confident and have a process to follow in order to answer the questions that inevitably come up with new drama therapy groups.

We definitely do not want anyone to use this book as a checklist. As Gary Klein says in his book about insights, "The downside of checklists is that they intentionally induce *mindlessness*. We just have to follow the steps and not think about them. The important thinking has been done by the checklist designers" (2013, p. 161, emphasis in the original). Each participant and each group that a drama therapist works with will be unique and will need their treatment plan and interventions to be created with detail, sensitivity, and critical thinking. We see this book as a map to keep you on the right path so you can make good choices.

We also definitely do not want anyone to see this book as an intellectual critique of drama therapy or psychological theories. We are not teaching new knowledge, as much as teaching how to synthesize and use the knowledge that you already have. We see this book as a practical tool, not an intellectual discourse.

The Drama Therapy Decision Tree

Gut reactions, intuition, and spontaneity are important to drama therapists. They assist in understanding the individual and the group in the here and now, at the current level of embodiment and in the physical space in which the therapeutic work happens. However, drama therapists also need to be able to communicate verbally and concretely with participants and other professionals about their decision-making process. This book does not negate gut reactions, intuition, or spontaneity; its purpose is to focus on the verbal, cognitive explanations of the process so they can be shared before and after the fact.

The book follows a decision tree structure that takes the drama therapist on a step-by-step journey through a series of questions (see Appendix A). There are different styles of decision trees. This one is not a yes/no model. This one is divided into branches or decision categories that need to be addressed: diagnosis, phase of treatment, psychological distance, interventions, assessment, diversity, and ethics.

The drama therapy decision tree is not designed as a bag of techniques, a checklist, or a shortcut to treatment planning. Instead, the decision tree provides a global, integrated model for therapeutic decision-making. The questions posed on those branches guide the therapist to gathering the necessary information so well-thought-through clinical choices can be made.

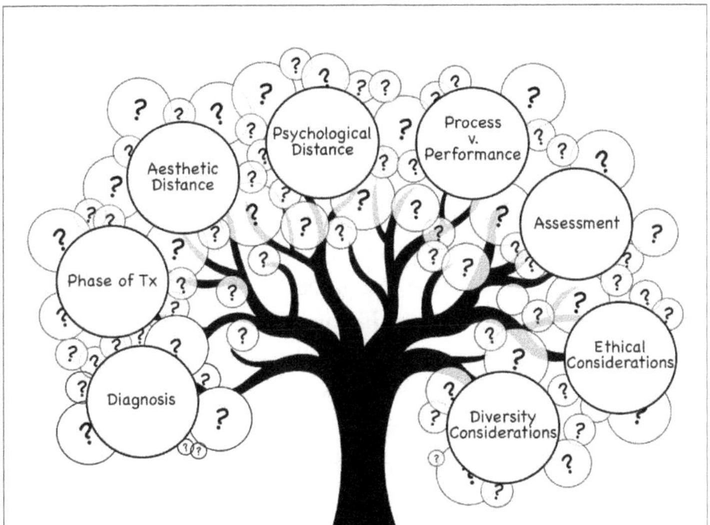

FIGURE 1: Drama Therapy Decision Tree. 2020. © Paige Dickinson and Sally Bailey. Infographic Design © Hunter Pressley.

The drama therapist is guided to break down complex clinical decisions into smaller components. For instance, the first part of the decision tree deals with the diagnosis of the individual, the specific symptoms being experienced, and the global functioning issues that have impacted their life.

Each question leads the drama therapist to gathering information that makes it possible to ask the next question in the decision-making process. These questions may at first seem to be overwhelming in number; however, they are all valid and necessary questions drama therapists need to ask themselves about participants at the beginning and throughout the process. They represent the list of questions that resulted after we reverse engineered the choices we consider consciously and unconsciously when we work with clients today. Using the drama therapy decision tree, students and early career professionals are provided with a common process to follow and common language for communicating that process with each other and with professional colleagues from other disciplines.

The Drama Therapy Framework

Drama therapy does not use one framework (e.g., psychology) to explain the healing process of a second framework (e.g., drama/theatre). Rather, drama therapy is a framework that combines both psychological and dramatic processes to explain healing. In other words, drama therapy is the interwoven, interconnected discipline of psychological and dramatic processes.

Different drama therapists approach their practice through the lenses of different psychological subframeworks. The treatment plans they create and the drama therapy interventions and theories they choose are often filtered through the psychological theory they espouse. This can be related to a specific drama therapy method. For instance, narradrama is filtered through narrative theory, and role method is connected to the archetypes of Jungian theory.

Other drama therapists may use one specific psychotherapeutic lens with all drama therapy interventions they use. For instance, a drama therapist with a psychodynamic viewpoint may interpret what happens in drama therapy sessions based on participants' conscious and unconscious drives, while a drama therapist who uses a behavior therapy perspective may interpret what happens in their sessions based on reinforcement and observational learning.

The drama therapy decision tree works for both approaches. The questions that a drama therapist must answer remain the same. The tree also allows for other mental health practitioners to better understand the choices that their drama therapy colleague is making.

Terminology Used in the Book

There are a number of terms used by more than one profession. Each has a different meaning or connotation for the professionals who use them. This is true even within the drama therapy field. For clarity, we are sharing the way in which we have defined the terms used in this book.

Drama Therapy Intervention

We are using the term *drama therapy intervention* for any method, approach, activity, game, technique, or exercise done for therapeutic reasons in a drama therapy session. Many times, drama therapists who come from theatre or education worlds call an activity a *theatre game*. Both Viola Spolin (1963), the mother of American improvisation, and Augusto Boal (1992), the Brazilian theatre director who created the theatre of the oppressed, used this term. For them the term *theatre game* had a very positive connotation, indicating playfulness and spontaneity, qualities valued in the theatre for breaking down actor inhibitions. However, the word *game* is often looked down on outside of theatre, because to most adults it connotes something trivial, which only children do. Recreational therapists often use the word *activity*, and for them this connotes something related to a daily living skill or an arts and crafts project. However, to the general public the word *activity* can connote an action that is mindless or unimportant.

Method is often used to refer to the theory and techniques developed by a specific drama therapist. For instance, Jacob Moreno created the techniques of role taking, role reversal, the double, and the empty chair to be used in his psychodrama and sociodrama methods. However, the term *method* can cause confusion as the words *technique* and *method* are often used interchangeably. In order to avoid this confusion, a text entitled *Current Approaches to Drama Therapy* (Emunah & Johnson, 2009; Lewis & Johnson, 2000), substituted the word *approach* for *method*. In counseling professions, the word *approach* is often used interchangeably for *theory* or *theoretical model*. The general public uses *approach* in a very generalized manner.

Hence, *intervention* will be used as an inclusive term for all endeavors undertaken in a drama therapy session. Using this word clearly indicates the intentionality of the drama therapist's choices for the work being done in the session.

Participant Versus Client Versus Consumer Versus Patient Versus Actor

In this book the words *participant, client, consumer, patient,* or *actor* are used based on the physical location of the drama therapy work: *actor* within a theatre or theatre education context, *patient* within a medical facility, *consumer* within a service organization, *client* within a mental health facility, and *participant* in a research capacity, in community-based programming, or when the location is unknown. While all these terms will be used, *participant* and *actor* will be used most often for a person involved in drama therapy interventions, because it seems less pathologizing.

Processing

Processing is the act of discussing an intervention by participant(s) and therapist about what the participant experienced, learned, is curious about, or been confused by during an intervention. Processing allows participants to notice the reaction of the therapist and others in the group and understand how their experience and reaction differs. Processing has the connotation of experiencing, meaning-making, insight, and integration which are the tasks of healing. The terms *discussion, talk, reflection,* and *processing* can be considered synonyms in this book.

Process-Oriented

Process-oriented is the way in which theatre professionals look at drama activities that lead to preparing an actor for a performance. Theatre educators talk about the difference between the *process* and the *product.* Drama therapists make a distinction between interventions that are done just within the group for the group with no intention of a future formal performance as *process-oriented* and rehearsing for a play as *presentation-oriented.* The other way that drama therapists look at *process-oriented* is that processing is a necessary component of some interventions versus interventions that can stand on their own. For example, psychodrama and sociodrama would be considered *process-oriented* intervention as they include a sharing at the end of the enactment.

Therapy Versus Therapeutic

An intervention is considered to be *therapy* if there is intent for change and/or relief and/or healing guided by a trained professional. An intervention is considered to be *therapeutic* when there is no intent for healing or change, but a positive change occurs anyway as a side effect. For example, acting in a play can be therapeutic for an actor. The actor can explore emotions and have a cathartic release. The cast of a play may become so close during the process of rehearsals and performance that they feel like a family, healing some of the rifts that actors may have in their family of origin. However, neither of these healing experiences happened intentionally; they happened as a side effect of being a part of a theatrical experience.

Self-revelatory performance is a form of therapy because a participant is guided by a drama therapist to create an original play that explores personal issues in order to bring closure and acceptance of them through rehearsal, performance, and the active witnessing of the audience. Without a drama therapist to guide this process, it is not *therapy;* it is a one-person or autobiographical play (Emunah, 2020; Pendzik, Emunah, & Johnson, 2016).

In educational theatre projects, there can be confusion between what is *therapy* and what is *therapeutic*, because in providing appropriate developmental and aesthetic education, socio-emotional learning and change often happen. Educational theatre is not therapy. The purpose of educational theatre is to teach students theatre skills and appreciation or to teach other academic subjects through theatre techniques. Drama therapists use the medium of a play to intentionally create change and promote healing in the actors who are acting in a play. An example of this would be barrier-free theatre (Bailey, 2010). A group of adults with and without disabilities work together to create an original play based on their ideas and improvisations. The intention is to teach social skills, emotional tolerance, executive functioning, emotional regulation, behavioral regulation, and self-expression through the process of developing and performing a play. The drama therapist gives thought to the individual and group needs of the actors and makes therapeutic and artistic decisions based on those needs. A theatre artist could follow a similar model of devising theatre with a group of people with disabilities, but they would not be trained to address the psychological, social, and physical needs of the actors.

By the same token an applied theatre method, such as the theatre of the oppressed or playback theatre, can be focused on revealing and exploring a social injustice or community issue. However, if it is not being used intentionally by a trained drama therapist as a healing technique for an identified client or client group, then it is not therapy. Drama therapist Armand Volkas (2009) has created a drama therapy intervention called healing the wounds of history. He uses sociodrama and playback theatre to help groups of people who have traditionally been enemies share their experiences with each other to break down the barriers of hatred. He has worked with groups of Germans and Jews, Chinese and Japanese, and Israelis and Palestinians to create understanding and healing. In these cases, he is using applied theatre techniques for drama therapy purposes.

One of the difficulties within applied theatre is the lack of ethical guidelines to help practitioners understand their boundaries and the scope of practice. A few applied theatre professionals go as far as claiming their work to be *therapy* because the "facilitator is in the role of the therapist and the participant is the patient"

(Prentki, 2016, p.15). Crossing this boundary can be dangerous as the applied theatre facilitator has not received the appropriate training in psychology, psychotherapy, or ethics to keep the participant safe. For applied theatre artists, we recommend you read "Generating Ethics and Social Justice in Applied Theatre Curricula" by Bailey and Dickinson in *New Directions in Teaching Theatre Arts* (2018).

Structure of the Book

This book is broken up into three sections. *Section One: Foundations* consists of three chapters. Chapter One, 'Foundational Principles of the Therapeutic Process,' addresses the foundational principles of individual and group psychotherapy processes and Renee Emunah's Five Phase Integrated Model of Drama Therapy. Chapter Two, 'Foundational Principles of Drama Therapy,' presents the core concepts of drama therapy and introduces the drama therapy pie. Chapter Three, 'Foundations of Diagnoses and Global Functioning,' discusses the DSM-5 and ICD-11, the internationally accepted manuals for diagnostic criteria. Other diagnostic concerns such as aspects of global functioning are also discussed.

Section Two: The Drama Therapy Decision Tree comprises three chapters. Chapter Four, 'A Systematic Method for Drama Therapy Treatment Planning,' explains how a treatment plan is created from a diagnosis. A fictional participant is used to demonstrate the kinds of questions needed to be answered to determine the goals and objectives of an individual treatment plan. Chapter Five, 'A Systematic Method for Choosing Drama Therapy Interventions,' guides the drama therapist in deciding which interventions should be used with specific participants or groups. Chapter Six, 'A Systematic Method for Drama Therapy Treatment Evaluation,' presents Susana Pendzik's six-key model that can be used for evaluating when goals and objectives have been successfully achieved with a participant and when it is time to create new objectives and goals.

Section Three: Diversity and Ethical Considerations consists of two chapters. Chapter Seven, 'Diversity: Cultural Competence, Adaptations, and Accommodations,' identifies concerns that clinicians need to be cognizant of in terms of diversity, cultural competency, and cultural humility. Information about adaptations and/or accommodations for participants who are of a different culture or who are differently abled are highlighted. Chapter Eight, 'Ethics,' provides questions to help drama therapists discern ethical dilemmas that might arise in relation to the choice of drama therapy interventions. These two chapters are only a brief overview of the major diversity and ethical issues that could arise; each chapter could be developed into a book on its own.

Conclusion

This book is a practical guide, not a checklist. Rather than using a standardized protocol that makes the decisions for the therapist, drama therapy is based on dynamic, embodied, creative action with participants in the here and now. Conscious planning on the part of the drama therapist before the session supports spontaneity and creativity, providing the information needed to make good therapeutic decisions in the moment during the session. The drama therapy decision tree is meant to be a tool for conscious planning and communication.

SECTION 1

FOUNDATIONS

1

Foundational Principles of the Therapeutic Process

There are no new ideas. All knowledge is built on the thoughts, experiences, and experiments of the practitioners that came before. The drama therapy decision tree is built on theories and philosophies that originate from theatre, psychology, psychotherapy, and drama therapy. Within and across these disciplines, ideas overlap, complement, and are integrated with each other. Each of the following foundational principles in Chapters 1, 2, and 3 have been integrated to create the drama therapy decision tree. Before presenting the decision tree, the authors believe that each of the foundational principles need to be understood and appreciated for what they contribute. This chapter focuses on the principles and processes of individual and group therapy. There are many similarities between an individual therapeutic process and a group one; however, because there are some differences, they will be discussed separately. In later chapters, as the book unfolds, how each set of principles is used will become apparent.

Individual Therapeutic Process Model

The individual therapy process does not originate from one specific theorist. Most textbooks divide the process into four stages; a few theorists divide it into five (Brammer & MacDonald, 2003; Egan, 2013; Okun & Kantrowitz, 2015). For clarity's sake, five will be identified here.

Intake/Assessment

The initial step of treatment is focused on the therapist getting to know the individual and building the therapeutic relationship. Often there is an intake form that guides the questions asked in the first session. The first session can also include a series of assessments. In certain environments, such as private practice, assessment and intake forms may not be as formal, allowing the therapist to ask open-ended questions. During the assessment the therapist collects two types of information: symptoms and dysfunctions. The therapist wants to explore why the individual is seeking treatment and what type of symptoms have been experienced. Gathering symptom information tends to be related to diagnosis of a particular problem, whereas identifying dysfunctions focuses on what problems the person feels are burdens. Sometimes these are the same, and sometimes they are different. Symptoms are important because labeling them leads to insurance approval, so sessions can be paid for. However, exploring what the participant believes is the most important issue can help build the therapeutic relationship and pinpoint what might need to be addressed first in treatment.

Research has shown that as much as one-third of the healing factors of therapy come from the therapeutic relationship (Miller, Duncan, & Hubble, 1997). An early part of the therapeutic relationship involves creating a safe environment by setting up the rules of treatment: cost, cancellation policies, informed consent, boundaries, and other rights and responsibilities of the participant. Another part is the verbal and nonverbal behavior of the therapist that helps the participant understand that empathy, listening, and engagement in the participant's problems are genuine.

Exploration/Goal Planning

During this stage the therapist and participant explore what they are going to work on in the therapeutic process. Together they examine patterns and identify specific emotional, behavioral, or cognitive changes that the participant wants to make. Once the exploration has started, they can define specific goals that can create change. During this stage the theoretical orientation of the therapist comes into play. For example, a therapist who comes from a cognitive-behavioral background may set detailed objectives about certain thoughts the participant needs to dispute, in order to change thinking and behavior, in order to meet the therapeutic goals.

Action Plan/Working

The majority of the therapeutic work is accomplished in this stage. This is also when resistance, transference, and other defense mechanisms can arise to interfere with the process. This happens not because the participant does not want to change, but because of the participant's fear of the unknown. If trust has been developed between the therapist and participant, these obstacles to moving forward in the change process can be dealt with successfully.

Reflection/Connection

This stage is sometimes combined with or split between stages three and five. The focus of this stage is reflecting on the work that has been done and on any adjustments that need to be made in order to reach the therapy goals. During this stage the participant begins to make connections between the work done in therapy and life. Time is also spent reflecting on the meaning of the relationship that has developed with the therapist. The therapist can become a re-parenting figure for the participant as past wounds are healed.

Termination

This can be a difficult stage for the participant and the therapist, because the relationship must come to an end. The therapist must handle this parting without making the participant feel abandoned. The participant needs to be able to verbalize what has been accomplished and what work needs to continue as therapy ends. A plan needs to be in place for what the participant should do if difficulties arise in the future. For someone with an addiction, this would be called a *relapse prevention plan.* For someone who had been sexually abused or depressed, it could be called a *safety plan.* Lastly, but most importantly, actually saying good-bye needs to be done. In Western culture many relationships are not terminated in a formal way; endings tend to be avoided because they feel uncomfortable. Respect and value are shown to a participant when the therapist takes the time to say good-bye in a genuine, therapeutic manner.

Irvin Yalom's Theory and Practice of Group Psychotherapy

One of the foundational theorists for group psychotherapy is Irvin Yalom. Yalom identified a number of core concepts of group development that all groups go through to create cohesion and functionality (Yalom & Leszcz, 2005). His ideas are in alignment with any therapeutic process no matter the theoretical outlook. Yalom is not studied directly in drama therapy courses, and we feel he should be. Through careful observation and thought about his therapeutic groups and those of other practitioners, he identified a pattern of group development that appears to be universal (see Figure 2).

COMPARISON: MODELS OF GROUP DEVELOPMENT

Yalom's 5 Stage Model (2005)	Emunah's 5 Phase Model (1994)	Hartford (1972)	Northen (1969)	Tuckman (1965)
Stage 1: Orientation	Phase 1: Play	Formation	Orientation	Forming
Stage 2: Conflict	Phase 2: Scene Work	Integration Disintegration and Reintegration	Exploration and Testing	Storming
Stage 3: Cohesiveness	Phase 3: Role-Play		Problem-Solving	Norming
Stage 4: Working	Phase 4: Culminating Enactments	Group Functioning & Maintenance		Performing
Stage 5: Terminating	Phase 5: Dramatic Ritual	Termination	Termination	Adjourning

FIGURE 2: Comparison Chart: The Stages of Group Process. 2000. © Sally Bailey.

His model of group development consists of five stages: orientation, conflict, cohesiveness, working, and termination.

Stages of Group Development

Stage One: Orientation

The therapist's role is in the spotlight during stage one because the group looks to the leader to set up the purpose of the group and provide the rules and norms by which everyone will abide. The therapist is a model of how to behave, so the group is shown, rather than told, what is expected of them. If the therapist is not willing to "walk the walk," the group members may not feel compelled to either and can lose respect for the therapist as the one in charge.

Group members in this stage tend to be guarded, because they do not trust each other, the therapist, or the process yet. This is particularly true for first-time participants who have never been in a therapy group. Often group members will be fearful of revealing their true selves for fear of criticism and humiliation. Sometimes they deflect from the issues of the group to complain about outside situations over which they have little control, such as the weather, the state of neighborhood schools, or the displacement of refugees.

Defensive and *resistant* are the traditional terms used for group members who refuse to participate or remain critical and remote. A good therapist expects this at the beginning as a natural reaction and must find ways to engage group members. Trust must be developed, as well as a belief in the group as a safe place to explore psychological issues. If a therapist responds to resistance by fighting it, often more resistance is created. Therapists can develop their own style of engaging resistant participants through careful warm-up, humor, playful challenge, and showing genuine interest.

In this first stage, group members are exploring the roles they will take on in the group. Will they be leaders or followers? Will they jump into activities and discussions fully or just dip their toes in the water? Will they connect deeply with the others in the group, or will they continue to hold back from personal intimacy?

When the group is ready to move to the next stage, the therapist will notice that the group members have accepted and are following the group rules and norms; they have begun to develop trust with each other and report feeling safe, and interactions among group members have become more open, respectful, and caring.

Stage Two: Conflict

The therapist continues to be a role model to demonstrate to participants how to self-disclose, how to be genuine and real, and how to talk in concrete and concise ways, rather than in vague abstractions or disorganized meanderings. Once participants have shared their general story, the therapist asks pointed questions to probe into more specific details. While group members know the purpose of the group at this point, they can still be inconsistent in their behavior. They may react to the therapist's push for more disclosure by creating conflicts between members to distract from the issues or by alternating between open self-disclosure and holding back. They may test boundaries to see if the therapist will hold firm on the rules and regulations. Sometimes they will be willing to listen to others, but if they feel uncomfortable or crave attention, they could block others or respond inappropriately. In short, they are still building the skills necessary to become a productive, effective therapy group. If the therapist continues to model appropriate interaction behavior and skillfully intervenes when group members are ignoring the rules, the group matures.

The therapist knows the group is ready to move to stage three when members begin reporting that they feel closer to their fellow participants. Verbal and nonverbal reactions become more respectful, sensitive, and thoughtful.

More group members demonstrate the willingness to take risks in terms of sharing personal struggles.

Stage Three: Cohesiveness

In this stage, group members have become close enough to share willingly. However, if one participant is not being honest or respectful, the rest will tend to avoid confrontation. Psychotherapeutic work slows down when all are on their best behavior and wait for the therapist to intervene. While this can be frustrating for the therapist who wants to forge ahead, the work of this stage must focus on its name: creating cohesion in the group before moving to deeper levels in stage four. If time is not spent on the creation of bonds among the group members, relationships will fall apart when the work begins to deepen later. The therapist knows the group is ready to move to the next stage when conflict has receded, confrontation is appropriate when it happens, cohesion is solid, and members are showing genuine emotional attachments.

Stage Four: Working

At stage four, group members will have internalized the rules, norms, and purposes of the group and know how to function within them. Ideally, they become more active than the therapist and are even able to set goals for the group. This does not mean that therapists sit back and put their feet up; they need to continue to keep the group on track by modeling how to confront and pointing out discrepancies and dissonances that group members may be missing or may not have the courage to address. At this stage participants are ready to change and willing to hold each other accountable to their commitment to change. Participants can mutually aid each other through support, empathy, listening, sharing ideas, and teaching each other skills.

In the best of all possible worlds, participants would remain in stage four until all of their issues were resolved, but this is unrealistic. The therapist may intuit that the work of the group has progressed enough so that staying together longer would create stagnation. More often the fourth stage may need to give way to the fifth stage because the number of sessions that were approved for the group by insurance or grant funding are coming to an end.

Stage Five: Termination

There are many reasons for termination. Currently, most groups are time limited. In this situation, several sessions before the final meeting, the therapist must move the group into the work of closure or termination. In a group that is not time limited, indications that the group is ready to terminate is when participants have developed the ability to practice their discoveries and insights outside of the group, experience a certain amount of success (or make adaptations for behaviors that did not quite work), and understand the changes they have made.

Ambivalence in the behavior and attitudes of group members often returns as the end of the therapy series approaches. The job of the therapist in this stage is to validate and reinforce what the group members have identified and accomplished, so they are clearly aware of the distance they have traveled. Yalom stresses that when a group closes, feelings of grief and loss are experienced by participants and therapist alike. The more successful a group has been, the more feelings of loss there will be. The best way to address these feelings is to deal with them in a reflective and positive manner, sending participants out into the world with a sense of accomplishment and hope. Yalom feels that therapists need to address their feelings about termination as well.

Eleven Therapeutic Factors

Yalom and Leszcz (2005) have identified eleven therapeutic factors that help group members heal during the course of the therapeutic process: *installation of hope, universality, altruism, the corrective recapitulation of the primary family group, development of socializing techniques, imparting information, imitative behavior, interpersonal learning, group cohesiveness, catharsis,* and *existential factors*. These factors also relate to participants in individual therapy, but working in a group increases the effectiveness of the factors. These eleven therapeutic factors are ingredients that all therapists, no matter what their theoretical orientation, should include in their practice. Research has shown that the work that the participant does in therapy is responsible for 40 percent of improvement, and the psychotherapeutic relationship between the therapist and participant is responsible for about 30 percent, while the model and technique constitute only 15 percent. The last 15 percent is attributed to expectancy and hope (Miller et al., 1997).

Installation of Hope

Since hope is responsible for at least 15 percent of the improvement that happens during therapeutic work (Miller et al., 1997), it is appropriate that installation of hope is the first factor Yalom talks about in his classic book *The Theory and Practice of Group Psychotherapy* (Yalom & Leszcz, 2005). Therapeutic work is hard and often painful. In dark times of struggle, hope is the only thing that keeps a participant engaged: hope for the pain to go away, hope for connection to others, hope for the solution to problems to become apparent. Without hope in life, in positive possibilities for the future, there seems to be no reason to go on.

If participants do not have hope, the therapist has to hold the hope for them and believe in the effectiveness of the work that they will do together. In our respective practices, both authors have had participants say to us, "You believed in me when I didn't believe in myself. That kept me going. I didn't want to let you down." While it would be preferable for participants to hold onto hope themselves, projecting that hope into the therapist at least keeps it alive until such time as the participants can re-own it. In a group, especially one that is not yet cohesive, holding onto hope can be difficult for the therapist, but by holding on, hope is kept alive within the group. Think of hope as an action, not just a passive wish. Besides the ability to create a warm therapeutic relationship, the installation of hope may be the most important action a therapist can take.

Universality

Many participants come to therapy believing that no one will understand their suffering because no one is like them. This belief is a little naive and narcissistic; however, it expresses how isolated and hopeless the participant feels. Universality is the notion that all human beings share the human experience; therefore, we are not alone, and we are not the only one suffering from a specific problem. Because that is true, others—the therapist and the group members—can understand us. When participants understand their problems are universal, they can often relax in the knowledge that if others have overcome their difficulties, perhaps they can too.

Altruism

In groups, as in life, we receive through giving—support, reassurance, insights, suggestions, even confrontation. Altruism involves giving without the expectation of receiving in return, giving because the giver genuinely cares about the receiver and is not thinking about self. There are no strings attached in altruistic giving and no hidden agendas. Experiencing freely given emotional offers can be very healing for participants who have grown up in families where every favor required a mandatory favor in return. In addition, group members often find it easier to accept information from peers than from the therapist or an authority figure. Giving to others also creates a connection between people and allows them to feel less isolated.

The Corrective Recapitulation of the Primary Family Group

At different points during the therapeutic process, members of the group metaphorically take on the roles of family members in each other's family of origin, but in a healthy, functional manner. For instance, in one session Fred could provide Tucker with the maternal, unconditional understanding that a mother might give or the rousing support and admiration that a father might offer. Through reexperiencing those relationships in a positive way, the deficits that were in the original family dynamics can be healed.

The healing can go both ways. Fred might have needed that kind of support from his father, but did not get it. In taking on the role of a functional father, Fred can experience what that supporting action feels like. Altruism comes into this corrective recapitulation, as the exchange of healthy interactions is a gift to both people.

Family reenactment happens in individual therapy with the therapist reenacting the different family roles (metaphorically speaking); however, there are more people available to play family roles in a group. Through these interactions new behaviors and relationships can be tested and practiced. (In a drama therapy group, group members can actually play the roles of real or fictional family members in dramatized scenes. This allows dialogues to develop, which either heal old wounds or provide practice for future boundary setting.)

Development of Socializing Techniques

This therapeutic factor refers to learning social skills through the modeling of appropriate behavior by the therapist and other group members. This can happen through interactive group dialogue as participants learn how to listen actively and deeply to each other and to share time in the spotlight. Practicing social skills through role-play allows group members to rehearse difficult interactions like assertiveness or apology.

Imparting Information

Imparting information refers to the direct guidance provided by the therapist and other members of the group. On the therapist's part, this includes the rules and norms of the group and whatever psychoeducation is necessary for the participants to understand their obstacles. For instance, in a group working on issues of disordered eating, there are facts about nutrition, statistics about different types of disordered eating, its effects on health, and so on that need to be shared. However, the information provided by the therapist is not as valuable as allowing the participants to discover and share the information themselves. When this is done, the therapist can step in to clarify, make the implicit explicit, or provide concretizing examples for abstract information.

Imparting information is not giving advice. Giving advice by a therapist or group member will not benefit the therapeutic process. Implicit in giving advice is a one-up power position taken by the advice giver, expressed sometimes as condescension and sometimes as sympathy. However, there can be indirect benefits if a participant gives advice because it demonstrates care and concern to the recipient. The advice giver may have similar problems and need an opportunity to formulate those answers.

Imitative Behavior

In individual therapy the participant often imitates the therapist, but in group therapy there are more people to model. This is often underestimated in terms of its importance. Vicarious learning can be more powerful than direct didactic imparting of information. Group members can try on the new behaviors they see in others to test them out. Scenes that are enacted in a drama therapy group offer additional behaviors that, if effective, could be imitated.

Interpersonal Learning

A therapy group is a microcosm of society. In the beginning, it might be as stressful and chaotic a microcosm as the participants' real lives are, but as the group matures over time, it can become a prototype of a more functional, possible world. Through socializing techniques, imitative behavior, and interpersonal learning, the participants practice better ways of interacting.

Sally Bailey's drama therapy groups at Second Genesis, a long-term residential drug rehabilitation program in the Washington, DC area, usually developed cohesion quickly. Even though her participants tended to be very self-centered and immature, the novelty and fun that drama therapy brought to the facility was very different from their usual confrontational groups. One day a group member challenged the rest of the group during the closure saying:

> This past week everybody has been so disrespectful, belligerent, and downright mean to each other. Why can't we treat each other the rest of the week like we treat each other in drama group? We are best friends here—brothers and sisters—but we leave this room and we start picking at each other. Why do we do that?

It was a moment of insight for himself and the rest of the group. They realized that they had the ability to be more civil to each other and work together cooperatively, but during the week they had been acting out old habits they had developed when they were in prison or out on the streets doing drugs.

A large part of interpersonal learning relates to the development of interpersonal relationships. Human beings are social animals. Interpersonal relationships are essential for survival. The attachments that form between mother and child are the beginnings of interpersonal relationships, which then branch out to other significant others and continue throughout our lifetimes. When we are not connected to others, our lives become unbalanced and lonely. Anxiety, loneliness, and depression can develop, and many studies have shown that this leads to illness, unhappiness, and early death (Ma et al., 2019). A therapeutic group provides the space for modifying interpersonal dysfunctions.

Corrective emotional experience develops as participants are exposed to group situations during which they recognize their negative projective defenses have become habitual behavior: rebelling against authority figures as if they were an abusive father or replaying the pecking order of sibling rivalry. Beyond cognitively recognizing these poor relational habits, mistakes must be felt before a behavioral correction can be substituted; otherwise, there will be no motivation for change. When the group learns how to function well, all the members can behave as their true selves, accepted by and relating to others in healthy, genuine ways.

Obvious maladaptive social patterns come to the surface in the beginning phases of the group. Subtler maladaptive patterns, such as hidden agendas, exploitation or manipulation of others, and disengagement from intimacy, can appear in later stages. The therapist can address these behaviors through the interactions of the group and through therapeutic interventions.

Group Cohesiveness

Group cohesiveness "refers to the attraction that members have for their group and the other members" (Yalom & Leszcz, 2005, p. 75). Cohesive group members are accepting and supportive of one another, inclined to form meaningful relationships, and willing to express and explore themselves. A cohesive group will have more participation, listening, and sharing going on among the members. There are trusting relationships between the participants and therapist and among group members. Communication within the group is direct and open. When appropriate, participants can confront each other. The strong connections that exist among them allow group members to express negative feelings without fear that their relationship will fall apart.

Catharsis

Yalom defines catharsis as the release of emotional experience and expression, both positive and negative. He believes it is necessary for affect to be released. However, just having a moment of catharsis is not enough; there must also be insight and behavior change to go along with it. Emotion for emotion's sake is a waste of time. Catharsis is not necessarily the result when a participant breaks down in tears. The emotional expression of catharsis can be tears, laughter, or another intense response. In addition to the intensity of the emotion, the expression must be genuine and related to the psychotherapeutic work being done. This way of defining catharsis is important because there are highly emotional people who cry easily and like to garner attention in groups by working themselves up to a state of tears. This is emotional flooding or manipulation, not catharsis.

Existential Factors

Existential factors consist of:

1. Recognizing that life is at times unfair and unjust.
2. Recognizing that ultimately there is no escape from some of life's pain or from death.
3. Recognizing that no matter how close I get to other people, I must still face life alone.
4. Facing the basic issues of my life and death, and thus living my life more honestly and being less caught up in trivialities.
5. Learning that I must take ultimate responsibility for the way I live my life no matter how much guidance and support I get from others.

(Yalom & Leszcz, 2005, p. 98)

No one can escape responsibility, isolation, mortality, honesty, and accepting the consequences for their choices. These five factors are a crucial part of the group process, no matter what theoretical orientation is followed.

Renee Emunah and the Integrative Five-Phase Model of Drama Therapy

The integrative five-phase model of drama therapy was developed by Renee Emunah (2020) based on her drama therapy experiences with participants over many years. It overlays drama therapy theories and techniques on top of traditional group development processes. Like Yalom and other group development theorists (see Figure 2), Emunah has conceptualized the evolution of groups over time to assist drama therapists in understanding the type of drama therapy interventions that are appropriate for the group dynamics and the current level of therapeutic growth of the participants.

Phase One: Dramatic Play

Phase one focuses on the introduction of the participants to each other, the therapist, and the basics of drama therapy. From the first session, the groundwork is laid for play: social games, drama games, dramatic play, and beginning improvisation. Participants, who may not have played since grade school, are invited to engage with each other, free themselves from their inhibitions in a nonthreatening environment, and have fun. The focus is on the group playing together, not on solo performance, so no one needs to worry about being put on the spot or put in the spotlight until they are ready. Team building is the focus. Individuals, who have become rigid in terms of interactions with others, learn to relax and connect. Through play, group members also learn flexibility, fluidity, and spontaneity.

In phase one there is just enough structure through the use of theatre games and other interventions for participants to feel comfortable enough to enter into the playspace, begin to trust each other, and learn basic, appropriate, interactive behavior. Setting the rules and norms for drama in this active environment prepares participants for later phases of treatment. Just as in Yalom's group model, Emunah encourages drama therapists to start the process of guiding their participants toward openness, acceptance, and understanding from the very beginning of the work. Participants who have difficulty following rules learn the importance of rules for creating a satisfying and safe group experience. Participants who are shy or have anxiety begin to develop social relatedness. Participants who are rigid and inflexible begin learning give-and-take, cooperation, and how to share.

Humans seem to be biologically wired to play, just as we are biologically wired to learn language (Brown & Vaughn, 2009). Dramatic play is one of our innate ways of learning (Brown & Vaughn, 2009; Vygotsky, 1978; Weininger, 1988). Between the ages of two-and-a-half and three, children move naturally from sensorimotor play to dramatic play (Brown & Vaughn, 2009). Piaget (Flavel, 1963) would call this stage *preoperational.* Vygotsky (1978) focused on the pretend role-playing that children engage in at this time, which he believed guides them to develop social skills, learn about the culture around them, and begin to move their external speech into internal speech or thought.

In Emunah's phase one participants practice entering into the playspace, the place where healing and change can happen (Emunah, 2020; Johnson, 1991).

In the next chapter the concept of dramatic reality (Susana Pendzik's term for the playspace) will be explored more fully. Because it is an imaginal space that we have inhabited before, we are able to reenter it and relearn to play.

Play is at the root of imagination, creativity, and the ability to think. In the process of playing we create metaphor and social connections (Brown & Vaughn, 2009). Dramatic play introduces the concept of *role*. When children play, they take on the roles of the adults they see around them (Mommy, Doctor, Baby) or characters in the stories they have heard or seen on video. By acting out these characters, they learn how to work with others to build a story and practice the actions they see happening around them. Through play, drama therapy participants take on different roles in a safe manner. This adds a layer of safety. Even though they are fictional, phase one roles allow the role-taker to practice new behaviors and begin to expand what drama therapists call *role repertoire* (Emunah, 2020). Role repertoire refers to the number of roles that an individual feels comfortable playing in life. Someone with a wide repertoire has more behaviors to choose from than someone with a small repertoire.

Russian theatre director and actor Constantin Stanislavski (1948) introduced the idea of the *magic if* to theatre exploration. The *magic if* permits actors to bring their imaginations to the lives of their characters in terms of history, attitudes, and thoughts so they can bring their role vividly to life. Child psychiatrist Otto Weininger (1988) built on Stanislavski's *magic if* and conceptualized imagination as the ability to pose questions and think about *what if?* and behave *as if*. In dramatic play, participants pretend *as if* they are someone else or use an object *as if* it is something else. In Weininger's model, imagination and pretend, while different processes, are intimately connected to and build on each other reciprocally. The ability to use the *as if* does not go away with age; it continues to be a skill we can access at any time. These skills are re-introduced and practiced in phase one.

Yalom and Leszcz (2005) say that resistance is present in the first stage of a group. In an early drama therapy group, resistance comes up, but is often dealt with through humor and play. Once participants start having fun and laughing together, resistance usually begins to melt away. It may not be totally gone; resistance may return later when participants are challenged to take a risk that reveals personal information. The resistance of phase one is more about hesitancy, fear of the unknown, and uncertainty, rather than fear of feeling emotions or fear of people knowing your uncomfortable secrets. Because of this, resistance can often be played with.

The transition from phase one to phase two is often a gentle progression from theatre games and improvisation to more structured improvisational scenes. Sometimes phase one and phase two overlap. This is in alignment with how Yalom and Leszcz (2005) see the changes from orientation to conflict.

Phase Two: Scenework

Emunah sees this phase as a transitional one as well. As they move into phase two, participants begin to learn how to sustain and develop characters through dialogue and nonverbal expressions like tone of voice, facial expression, and movement. "In the middle of Phase Two, the scenes typically take on greater depth and complexity, leading clients to feel naturally inclined to comment on their enactments" (Emunah, 2020, p. 10). This aligns with Yalom's and Leszcz's model (2005), as they observe that within stage two, participants are more willing to share information about themselves and make comments on what others have said. Participants are ready to transition from phase two to phase three when they begin voluntarily commenting on the life-drama connection about the scenes being enacted (more about the life-drama connection in Chapter Two). This is similar to the switch from Yalom's conflict stage to the cohesiveness stage, when participants become more willing to take risks and make connections, and by doing this, take on more responsibility for the work of the group (Yalom & Leszcz, 2005).

It is quite possible that a group with severe interpersonal deficits will need to stay in phase one and/or two for the duration of their time in drama therapy. The drama therapist should not move the group forward to the activities of the next phase if group members are not showing respect for each other and are not yet committed to the work. If a group is moved forward before they are ready, the drama therapist will experience resistance and distrust from the group. Anyone who does volunteer to work may be put on the spot or mocked by the unsupportive witnesses. Staying in phases one and/or two, however, does not mean that the drama therapist has failed. It means that the group needs to focus primarily on social skills, trust building, rule following, and respect. Dramatic play and scene work are perfect for working on these issues.

Talking about building group and drama skills, brings up the necessity of addressing the need for a closed group, if possible. No new members are added to a closed group after the first or second session. Adding new members might not be a huge problem in talk therapy groups, but in drama therapy it can be. Most adults tend to feel inhibited about getting out of their chairs and playing or performing with others. Bringing new people into a drama therapy group can disrupt the trust that has started to be built and create worries about judgment from strangers. Adding new members can work if the established group is mature enough to welcome the new member(s) and serve as role models for them. However, a large number of new members added after phase one can throw off the balance of the whole group, causing a need to reform norms. When this happens, the whole group regresses back to phase one.

Phase Three: Role-Play

Participants in this stage are willing to explore their relationships within the group, mirroring the behavior of participants in Yalom's cohesiveness stage. Scene work becomes more structured as group members act out role-plays based on real-life scenarios with fictional characters. Rehearsal for life takes on more seriousness. When Sally Bailey worked with recovering drug addicts at Second Genesis in Washington, DC, she would set up role-plays in phase three about issues that residents would face when they left the facility. In these scenes, they did not play themselves; they created a fictional character with a different name. Different people would volunteer to play the Recovering Addict on his way to an NA meeting in his home neighborhood, and others would play the Drug Dealer waiting at the corner. Each Recovering Addict had to try to avoid buying drugs from the Drug Dealer. Because they were not playing themselves, no one was put on the spot for making a mistake. This allowed the group to discuss very highly charged emotional situations with some distance. Care was taken not to trigger anyone. Practicing those new roles in drama therapy group makes it easier to enact them when they happen in real life. In fact, when Second Genesis residents came back from their first weekend passes, they would seek out Sally to tell her that they actually had met up with their old drug dealer on the way to an NA meeting, and they had used the techniques and words practiced in drama group. "And they worked!"

Just as Yalom talks about the installation of hope in the group process, Emunah (2020) speaks of phase three as being a time when participants begin to experience the hope that their behavior can change and that their lives can become different. In this phase, participants' role repertoires can start to expand, and their style of playing familiar roles can be deepened and diversified. The drama therapist knows that it is time to move from phase three into phase four when the cohesiveness of the group has gelled, and when empathy has grown to the point that members will support each other regardless of the content of the personal event being enacted.

Phase Four: Culminating Enactment

In this phase participants begin to address unresolved issues and negative behavior patterns that they have been unwilling or unable to deal with. Through nonfictional drama therapy techniques, such as psychodrama, playback, or the creation of autobiographical performances, participants engage in reparation of those dilemmas. Serious content can be worked on at this point because of the trust, respect, and caring that the group members feel for each other. As participants engage in these explorations, insight deepens, buried emotions come to the fore, and catharsis is experienced. While one person works on a personal issue, the rest of the group members participate as other characters in the scene and serve as witnesses. Participants learn how to express and experience more intense emotions, both while engaged in the drama and while watching it. The distinction between Emunah and Yalom, in relation to the fourth phase/stage of group development, is that Emunah is more focused on the depth and intensity of emotion, self-exposure, and release of traumatic content of the work done by participants, while Yalom is more concerned with participants' commitment to the work. Yalom would be as happy for a participant to work deeply on issues of procrastination that have blocked functioning in the world as he would their childhood trauma. Part of this difference in focus is made possible because of the practice participants have had in dramatic enactment and emotional expansion and containment (i.e., emotional regulation) in the prior three phases. Phase four of drama therapy allows participants to dive deeply and safely into emotional scenes and return.

Phase Five: Dramatic Ritual

The final phase allows participants to assimilate the changes they have made during the group process as they prepare to end their time in therapy. During this phase it is important to celebrate the work done, validate the growth and effort put into the work, and prepare to deal with feelings of loss and sadness that come up when a group that has developed a deep level of intimacy ends. Dramatic rituals provide a safe structure for closure. In addition, review and reflection through discussion ties loose ends together. Focus is put on participants leaving with successful treatment outcomes, with a feeling of hope and optimism for the future, and belief in the possibilities of what the world holds for them. Yalom mentions that resistance can resurface during the last stage of treatment; in Emunah's model dramatic rituals may contain and deal with the ambivalence and avoidance that participants may have to termination.

Conclusion

Irvin Yalom and Leszcz (2005), Renee Emunah (1994), and other theorists have identified the stages/phases that individuals and groups progress through in a constructive therapeutic process. These stages/phases need to be respected if therapy is to proceed smoothly, and resistance and other defenses are to be minimized. The actual therapy process, whether individual or group, talk therapy or drama therapy, has a natural progression that starts slowly in order to develop that most valuable therapeutic commodity: trust. When it is time to dive in, this allows the therapeutic work to be done in a deep manner. Once the end of the work comes, the participant must be able to recognize it, own it, and then more forward confidently.

The therapist cannot move stages around and do the third stage first and the second stage last, as if therapy were a play in the theatre of the absurd. If a therapist does that, participants will not feel safe, and their defenses will stop all forward progress. Worse, the participant may not come back to therapy. When drama therapy interventions are used, they must be matched with the phase the participants are in. Following Renee Emunah's five-phase model as a map to the drama therapy group process guides the drama therapist to make clear and appropriate decisions at the right times.

2

Foundational Principles of Drama Therapy

This chapter focuses on the building blocks of drama therapy. Taking stock of these components highlights many of the assets that add power to drama therapy interventions, above and beyond those inherent in group and individual psychotherapy processes that are centered on talk alone. First, Susana Pendzik (2006) has identified a primary core concept that is involved in all drama and drama therapy experiences. *Dramatic reality* represents the imaginary space in which drama therapy takes place. Second, Phil Jones (1996, 2007) has identified eight core concepts of drama therapy that can be found in all approaches and interventions of drama therapy. In other words, they are the raw materials out of which all drama therapy is built. Third, Sally Bailey's *drama therapy pie* (1999) models how all the various approaches and interventions used by drama therapists can be organized into a coherent system.

Susana Pendzik's Dramatic Reality

When engaging in dramatic play or creating a dramatic scene in theatre or therapy, actors temporarily suspend belief in the real world and enter into an imaginary world. While believing firmly in the imaginary world and pretending *as if* it is real and happening now (Stanislavski, 1948), actors do not become psychotic and lose touch with reality. A child knows she is not Rapunzel locked in a tower; she knows she is a girl standing on top of the slide in the backyard. An actor knows he is not Stanley Kowalski; he knows he is an actor on a theatre set. Human beings have the wonderful capability of being able to be in two places at once: the land of dramatic enactment and real life.

This concept has been called by many names: *surplus reality* (Moreno, 1959), *potential space* or *transitional space* (Winnicott, 1990), *the liminal field* (Blatner & Blatner, 1988), *the playspace* (Johnson, 1991), *the fictional present* (Cattanach, 1994), and *the aesthetic space* (Boal, 1993). However, drama therapist Susana Pendzik has done the best job of clearly defining the imaginary realm where drama and drama therapy takes place.

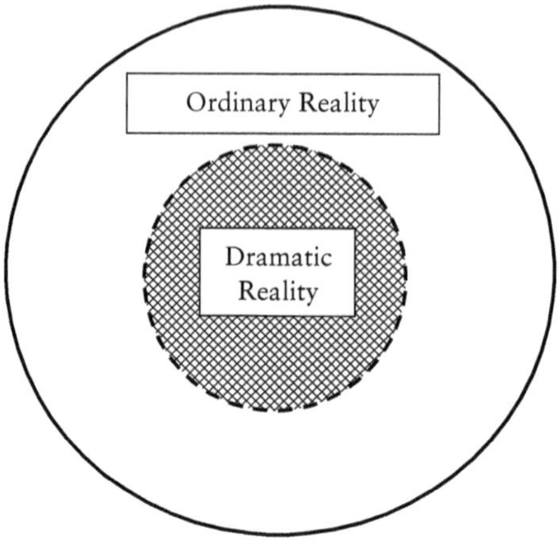

Reprinted from The Arts in Psychotherapy, Vol. 33, Susana Pendzik, On dramatic reality and its therapeutic function in drama therapy, Page 272, Copyright (2006), with permission from Elsevier.

FIGURE 3: Relationship of Dramatic Reality to Ordinary Reality. 2006. Infographic Design Susana Pendzik. © Elsevier Inc.

She calls it dramatic reality and has described its qualities and powers in depth (Pendzik 2003, 2006, 2008, 2012, 2018). She says, "Dramatic reality is imagination manifested," meaning the imagination is given form and substance whenever people create drama (2006, p. 272).

This diagram of dramatic reality shows that it is not separate from ordinary reality (see Figure 3). It is not literally in a different space or time; it is inside ordinary reality and real time. We can go there whenever we choose.

At the start of a drama therapy group, everyone enters the room in ordinary reality. When a drama game or scene starts, the players/actors enter dramatic reality. Group members who are watching the drama remain in ordinary reality, although they can choose to suspend their disbelief and be narratively transported into the story.[1] If the entire group is playing a game, everyone goes into dramatic reality. When the game or scene is done, the players return to ordinary reality and can talk about what they experienced.

Dramatic reality is a safe space into which personal feelings, ideas, relationships, and experiences can be projected (see dramatic projection in Phil Jones's core concepts). Dramatic reality then becomes a powerful space for therapy because all of those projected contents can be played within a "good arena for expressing difficult feelings, testing hypotheses, or reliving memories" (Pendzik, 2006, p. 273). The laws of dramatic reality are different from the laws of ordinary reality; they are the laws of the imagination. Time can be extended, sped up, slowed down, fast forwarded, rewound, or paused. Actions can be replayed to see what different consequences or feelings might result when other choices are made. Space can be transformed from one location to another in the blink of an eye with the agreement of the players. Dragons can be slayed and brought back to life. "In a world where everything is possible we are only bound by our own limitations and restrictions" (Pendzik, 2006, p. 273).

The job of the drama therapist is to help the participants make the transfer from ordinary reality to dramatic reality. For a warm-up game, the transfer might be as quick as getting into position, hearing a short description of the game, practicing a round, and jumping in. Sometimes the transition is prepared for through a discussion of what problems need to be explored in the playspace and how they might be addressed. Preparatory work can involve telling stories, writing poems, drawing maps, creating social atoms, or making pictures that will be dramatized.

There are participants who have more difficulty entering dramatic reality than others. This might be because it seems silly, scary, or embarrassing to explore one's life through embodied imagination. When drama is a new adult experience, the participant typically just needs practice in letting go of ordinary reality. All children between the ages of two and three naturally begin to do dramatic play, so everyone has had experience entering dramatic reality, and like riding a bicycle, it is easy to remember how. Usually, if participants are appropriately warmed up to make the transfer, they can easily slip into embodying a role and believing in the action of the scene. The drama therapist might remain outside in ordinary reality or might join the participants in dramatic reality as a guide, mentor, director, or supportive character. The drama therapist can side coach or stop the action of a scene to change the rules or the technique being used, thereby deepening the experience. For example, during a psychodrama or sociodrama the drama therapist can have actors reverse roles or double for each other. In any case, the drama therapist uses time in dramatic reality for making therapeutic interventions that facilitate participant insights.

Once back in ordinary reality at the conclusion of a scene, the drama therapist guides participants to reflect on their dramatized experiences and helps them make connections between what happened in dramatic reality and their own lives in ordinary reality, so they can integrate their insights. This is also the time to derole participants from the roles they enacted in the drama. Sometimes characters are easily left behind; in the bright light of ordinary reality, the imaginary world recedes. However, at other times when participants are playing themselves (as opposed to a fictional character), or have experienced intense emotions, more involved deroling rituals need to be done to step away from the role. More will be said about deroling in Chapter Five.

Susana Pendzik emphasizes:

> It is important to distinguish between *fantastic reality* (FR) and *dramatic reality* (DR) in drama therapy. In FR the locus of the *as if* is the imagination and in this sense, DR is an embodied form of FR. While FR can exist within a person's head (as in daydreaming or visualizing), DR manifests itself through actual form. FR *is* the invisible; DR is a concrete revelation of the invisible ... FR is the ignition of the engine, for without the capacity to imagine, to transcend into FR, there is nothing to channel into the ordinary world ... it is important to note the qualitative difference between imagination and its dramatic (action-oriented) manifestation. As Yanov (2012, 2014) claims, they probably involve different neurological processes and brain activity.
>
> (2018, pp. 189–190)

Phil Jones's Core Concepts of Drama Therapy

British dramatherapist Phil Jones (1996, 2007) identified eight core concepts that can be found in all drama therapy theories and interventions: *play, embodiment, dramatic projection, role-playing and personification, drama therapeutic empathy and distancing, active witnessing, the life-drama connection,* and *transformation.* These core concepts are all used in dramatic reality as building blocks for treatment. As he researched the core processes, he discovered that certain core processes become the center of attention in different sessions (2007). They should not be thought of as linear in relationship to each other or as functioning in a hierarchy. Instead, they are interwoven aspects that are part and parcel of every drama therapy session.

Play

Jones sees play as central to drama therapy practice (1996, 2007). Without play there can be no drama therapy because play is the fabric from which all drama therapy interventions are woven. Play engages participants in the group, enhances cohesion, and initiates spontaneity and the ability to stay in the here and now. Stodgy adults, who feel that anyone over the age of seven is too old to play, are unaware of the necessity of developmentally appropriate play throughout the life span. Play provides recreation and rest, enhances friendships and intimate relationships, and can be a helpful learning tool at any age (Brown & Vaughn, 2009).

Once group members embrace playing, they begin developing connections with their fellow group members, and they become willing to participate in other therapeutic activities. Play develops self-confidence, risk-taking, and curiosity; it makes the player feel alive again. Interviews with drama therapy participants revealed that

> play appeared to offer them a freedom that allowed them to engage with the playful parts of themselves. This in turn allowed them to bring feelings into awareness and acted as a vehicle for communicating to self and others.
> (Cassidy, Gumley, & Turnbull, 2017, p. 180)

Spinka, Newberry, and Bekoff (2001) define play as "training for the unexpected," which captures the essence of its value as a therapeutic tool. When a person can be spontaneous and present in the moment, they are better able to handle whatever obstacles are in their way. Playing teaches participants how to achieve that flexible state.

Current neuroscience indicates that play by animals and humans is crucial in brain development. Play rewires neural connections to allow the development of sensory integration (SI) and executive functioning (EF) (Brown & Vaughn, 2009; Pellis, Pellis, & Himmler, 2014). Often mental health dysfunctions can be traced back in part to poorly developed SI or EF. Sometimes this immaturity originates from organic neurological conditions like autism spectrum disorders (ASD) or attention deficit hyperactivity disorder (ADHD). However, dysfunctions can also originate from insufficient childhood play, which interferes with normal development. Children who have experienced abuse, abandonment, or neglect may have been unable to engage in normal play experiences. This later affects their abilities to socialize appropriately with peers. Perhaps they do not know how to inhibit inappropriate emotional responses and lose control when they do not get their way, or they may not be able to focus their attention on group tasks (Brown & Vaughn, 2009; Pellis et al., 2014). Beginning with play allows participants to experience a remedial social and emotional process necessary for connecting to and living successfully with others. Participants who do not need remedial help enjoy playing anyway.

Since play during normal development is necessary for growth, it stands to reason that play in therapy can jump-start growth that was previously delayed or denied. This is possible because of the brain's plasticity (Brown & Vaughn, 2009; Doidge, 2007; Pellis et al., 2014). Neurons continue to grow in many areas of the brain throughout the life span, meaning that deficits and damage can be repaired with appropriate interventions. For instance, stroke survivors often have brain damage where neurons have died from lack of oxygen. Physical therapy that requires them to use the parts of their body that were paralyzed can regenerate nerve networks and allow regrowth. If the parts of the brain that were directly affected by the stroke are beyond repair, then neurons in adjacent areas that are able can take over those actions (Doidge, 2007). Play interventions function in the same way for generating or regenerating parts of the brain necessary for self-regulation.

Embodiment

Embodiment is one of the aspects of drama therapy that distinguishes it from traditional talk therapy. It functions hand-in-hand with play. If they only sit and talk, participants miss out on experiential learning about themselves and others. Embodied experiences in drama therapy get participants out of their chairs and immerse them emotionally, cognitively, and physically in the action explorations undertaken in the group. The willingness of participants to embody their therapeutic investigations allow all of the other core processes of drama therapy to manifest in the session.

> The body, however, is not merely a vehicle for thoughts and feelings; it is the medium through which they are experienced and expressed. In forgetting this, we risk limiting our own expressive performance in many ways.
>
> (Duggan & Grainger, 1997, p. 125)

In the past 20 years the study of embodied cognition has exploded thanks to the ability to study the brain through positron emission tomography scans (PET), functional magnetic resonance imaging (fMRI), transcranial magnetic stimulation (TMS), and electroencephalogram testing (EEG). Research in Italy in the 1990s on the motor system in monkeys led to the discovery of the *mirror neuron system* (Gallese, Kesers, & Rizzolatti, 2004; Iacoboni et al., 2005). From there neuroscientists found connections between the sensory (perception) and motor (action) systems in the brain. So many connections were found that the two systems are now spoken of together as the *sensory-motor system*. Later links were discovered between the sensory-motor system and the language system; all are connected through the cerebellum to the frontal cortex (Gallese & Cuccio, 2018; Gallese & Lakoff, 2005; Kiefer & Trumpp, 2012).

Using a neural pathway for more than one purpose happens frequently as studies in neurobiology have shown. For instance, the circuits that carry messages about physical pain also carry messages about emotional pain (Williams, 2011). When a new internal process is developed, it makes evolutionary sense for a pathway that is already in existence to be used instead of creating a new one. This kind of efficient development creates better internal communication and a quicker ability to revise and adjust to sudden changes in the immediate environment, since the pathways connect instead of traveling in parallel circuits (Gallese & Cuccio, 2018; Gallese & Lakoff, 2005; Kiefer & Trumpp, 2012).

Cognition, then, does not just reside in the brain, but is also grounded in the body. Cognition is not separate from other brain functions like emotions and interior sensations (Damasio, 1994, 1999). The body brings experiences in through the senses and the muscles, explores the world through movement and emotion, and ultimately contributes to meaning-making as those experiences are processed in the frontal lobes of the brain.

Gerontology, nursing, and developmental psychology classes often include aging simulations as part of teaching students about an older adult's perspective. Educational research done on simulations have typically been qualitative studies about how students liked the simulation activity and if they had an "Aha" moment about what an aging person or a person with a disability experiences; however, the literature did not examine if these activities actually increased knowledge and understanding. To address that lack, Paige Dickinson, one of the authors, quantitatively examined if embodied activities increased knowledge and understanding (Dickinson, Schwartzmueller, & Martin, 2014). For this study, students took on one of two roles: an older adult or an adolescent. These characters were embodied and worked together. A third student served as a spotter with each team to ensure their safety. To get into role, each student was given a costume. The students playing older adults put on glasses that impaired vision, earplugs that hindered hearing, gloves that simulated loss of feeling in fingers from neuropathy and arthritis, small beads in their shoes to replicate loss of fatty tissue and neuropathy caused by diabetes, and after all that, they dressed in clothing with small buttons. The students playing adolescents took their shoes off and wore baggy clothes. They had an easier time getting into their role, being closer to the age of their characters. Each team was given a series of tasks to complete that took them around campus: they had to follow a map, read in a dimly lit room, practice short-term memory functions with a list of words, and complete an obstacle course. There was a time limit and incentives were offered for the first team to complete all the tasks. This gave the adolescent characters motivation to hurry the older adults along. The adolescents were also encouraged to say (in character) rude or insensitive things to their older adult partner that they had heard previously in public situations. After the activity, the students deroled: taking off their costumes, shaking out their bodies, and putting their own shoes and clothing back on. Students then discussed the activity. The control group (a different section of the class taught by the same instructor) learned about aging body changes only through a lecture.

Paige and her associates created an assessment instrument from several existing ones using the specifics of their aging simulation. The assessment was completed by students in the experimental class and the control class prior to the embodied activity and approximately two weeks after the activity. Results showed a significant increase in knowledge and understanding of the experiences of older adults from pretest to posttest in the experimental class in comparison to the control group. The control group showed no change from pretest to posttest. At the end of the semester, the control class's grades were lower than the experimental class by 10 percent in all units of the course. Not only did their embodied learning improve the experimental group's understanding of the unit, it seemed to positively affect their learning for the whole semester.

Dramatic Projection, Role-Playing, and Personification

Dramatic projection is the process of moving an idea, emotion, or thought from the mind of the individual into embodied action outside of the self. It can then be played with inside dramatic reality. This allows the internalization to be shared with the therapist and the group in a concrete, observable way. "Drama therapy involves downloading people's inner world into the physical realm of concrete forms" (Pendzik, 2018, p. 184). Dramatic projection builds on embodiment and allows the hidden to be seen. A dramatic projection could be concretized in a role, a puppet, a sculpt (human statue), a gesture, a sandtray figure, or a mask.

Role-playing and personification are aspects of dramatic projections, adding dialogue and movement as well as the creation of characters, embodied or projected. Through role-playing, reality can be explored to learn social problem-solving and how to function well with others under the rules of society. In the 1930s Russian psychologist Lev Vygotsky (1978) was a proponent of dramatic and make-believe play for children. He said that in play a child becomes "a head taller than himself," as he creates an imaginary situation, takes on and acts out roles, and practices following the rules of life which he has observed in the adult situations around him (Bodrova, Germeroth, & Leong, 2013; Vygotsky, 1978). Vygotsky believed that without dramatic play experiences, children would have difficulty understanding and developing social roles. They would not learn the rules of behavior or develop cultural competence, impulse control, and the symbolic manipulation of ideas (Bodrova & Leong, 2007; Vygotsky, 1978).

Improvisation and role-play, the adult forms of dramatic play, can perform the same function, allowing adults to rehearse for life. They learn how to function better within the rules of society: the social roles, behavioral expectations, cultural competencies, and emotional regulation required for success with others at work and at home. In some cases, drama therapy participants may need role-play to learn how to break out of the introjected, paralyzing, dysfunctional roles that they have been imprisoned in.

Vygotsky was not the only psychologist who saw play as a central component of healthy learning and growth. Otto Weininger (1988), also a developmental psychologist, conceptualized *imagination* as the ability to pose questions and think about *what if?* Following Stanislavski, he called *dramatic play* the experience of behaving *as if* one was someone else or using an object *as if* it was something else. He saw these actions as the beginning of the ability to imagine. In his model of development, imagining and pretending, which he saw as different processes, are intimately connected to and build on each other reciprocally.

The ability to use the *as if* does not go away with age; it continues to be a skill we can access at any time in our lives. Stanislavski used his acting method to teach actors how to develop their *as if* abilities to a fine degree (Stanislavski, 1948). Stanislavski's method continues to be used by contemporary actors. *As if* can also be applied to the classroom, the workplace, and the therapy group to assist in the invention of new skills, solutions to problems, or ways of interacting with others. The *as if* (what in theatre is termed *the willing suspension of disbelief*) provides a staging ground on which *what ifs* (imagination, ideas, images, or hypotheses) can be explored.

An interesting sidebar is a study done by Armstrong and colleagues (2016). The researchers created an operationalized definition for the core concepts of embodiment and dramatic projection. They analyzed each one by coding the behavior of a participant who was filmed doing drama therapy. Through their analysis, Armstrong and others confirmed that embodiment and dramatic projection are distinct processes and found that "drama therapy interventions involving dramatic embodiment may bring about sustained expression and processing, while dramatic projection interventions may have the opposite impact" (Armstrong et al., 2016, p. 30). This seems to indicate that embodiment is less distanced, and that dramatic projection is more distanced.

Empathy and Distancing

Jones sees empathy and distancing as connected concepts because they deal with the experience of the participants' emotions in the drama therapy session. Every psychologist who studies empathy has their own unique definition. Often empathy is confused with *sympathy*, an emotional reaction to someone else's experience involving pity or sorrow. Instead of an emotional reaction, empathy is the active engagement of trying to understand the emotional experience of another person. There are two types of empathy, both involve being able to "put oneself in the other's shoes," but they differ in quality. *Cognitive empathy* is a form of perspective taking or theory of mind. It focuses on being able to identify through reasoning what another person is feeling. *Affective empathy* allows one to vicariously feel what the other is feeling. Out of affective empathy can come concern and compassion for the other. The first is an embodied awareness and recognition of the other's state, while the second, because it is a felt, embodied experience, often leads to action (Harris, 2009). It is possible that the mirror neuron system is the neural basis from which empathy grows (Harris, 2009; Iacoboni et al., 2005; Shamay-Tsoory, Aharon-Peretz, & Perry, 2009). Empathetic response to others is the seed from which moral responses, friendships, loyalty, and pro-social behavior develop (Harris, 2009). Some participants who have experienced early neglect and trauma, personality disorders, or certain neurological conditions like ASD need to develop empathy so they can understand the experiences of others, not just their own. (More will be said about empathy in Chapter Three.)

Distancing relates to participants' emotional closeness to or distance from the dramatic experience. The closer the emotional involvement/less distanced participants are in an intervention, the less they can think about it and develop perspective and understanding. The more distanced the participants, the less emotionally involved they are. Participants, who are too close to the enacted material, can be flooded with emotion and become unable to function in the drama. At the opposite end of the spectrum, participants who are too distanced lose emotional connection and start to rationalize or "check out" of the drama. The optimum state is a balanced one called *aesthetic distance* (Scheff, 1979), where the participant is able to balance thinking and feeling in a dance that shifts back and forth between the two. As Scheff so succinctly puts it, aesthetic distance is when "both past distress and present safety are experienced equally and simultaneously" (1979, p. 96). The participant must be able to stay in the "here and now" while visiting or revisiting emotional experiences through drama. Insight is dependent upon being engaged enough to feel and distanced enough to think; this way meta-processing can happen and meaning can be made from the experience.

British dramatherapist Roger Grainger (2008) spoke of drama therapy as the purposeful manipulation of aesthetic distance, carried out to allow those involved the freedom to experiment with their own image of themselves, especially with regard to the crucial boundary between self and other. The ability to experiment is provided by the freedom that aesthetic distance gives participants. Grainger says, "The effect is to break the links which bind the present and past in the world outside, loosening their power to limit our freedom" (2008, p. 44).

Distance Considerations

There are two aspects of distancing that need to be examined with regard to drama therapy practice. First, the participant's *psychological distance* refers to participants' abilities to regulate their emotional responses. Second, *aesthetic distance* refers to the degree an intervention is able to evoke an emotional response versus a cognitive response. These two aspects of distance can be thought of as parallel continuums. Psychological distance can impact the aesthetic distance of the intervention. However, the intervention's place on the continuum can be harnessed to adjust the participant's psychological distance.

Psychological Distance of the Participant

Group members can be overdistanced or underdistanced in terms of their general personality style and in terms of the mood they are in at any given moment. In relation to general personality style, people who are generally overdistanced tend to exhibit signs of rigidity, lack of affect, and lack of connection to the therapist and others. They are caught in their thoughts and disconnected from their emotions. If you ask them how they feel, they might say "nothing," or they might tell you what they are thinking about, but not what they are feeling. In some cases, they cannot identify how they feel because they are not yet able to identify emotions by name. In other cases, they are so afraid to get in touch with their feelings that they consciously repress them or unconsciously suppress them.

People who are generally underdistanced tend to become easily emotionally flooded (i.e., experience inappropriate levels of emotional response). They are caught in their emotions most of the time and disconnected from their cognition. To have and remember insights, a person needs to be in a state of balance in which emotion and cognition coexist or, in other words, where emotional regulation allows one to have cognitive insight as well as feeling.

Beyond the personality style, there are days when anyone can arrive at the group overly emotional or very disconnected. They may have had a horrible day. They may be stunned by a sudden loss in their family or by a local, national, or international disaster. They may feel guilty because they did not complete an assignment for the group or had a relapse of some kind since the last meeting. If the therapist does not make an adjustment in their psychological distance, they will not get very much out of the group.

Many participants are in therapy because they have poor emotional regulation skills. They might not know how to readjust their attitudes before coming into the drama group, at least not in the early phases. The therapist has to show them how to readjust and regulate themselves through the interventions used. At one point, Sally was going from one Second Genesis facility to another to do a weekly drama therapy group. She often entered a facility and knew immediately from the atmosphere that something negative had gone on since the last time she was there. She needed to check in with staff to find out what had happened. During times when the atmosphere was intense, residents showed up to the drama therapy group sullen and resistant. Quite frequently what she had planned to do for warm-up had to be thrown out the window and replaced with one of several warm-ups that could be relied upon to turn bad moods into open, relaxed, attentive moods.

Aesthetic Distance of the Intervention

Drama therapy interventions inherently create specific amounts of distance. An intervention with more inherent distance will evoke less intense emotions either through the amount of embodiment versus projection, through the amount of emotion versus thinking engaged, or the amount of fiction versus nonfiction involved. Examples of interventions that typically have more distance are puppets, many drama games, and sociodrama. Interventions with less distance, tend to involve the body more and arouse more intense emotions. Examples of interventions with less distance would be psychodrama and developmental transformations (DvT).

Active Witnessing

In any form of therapy, the therapist is witness to the participant and the participant's story. In group therapy, group members are also witnesses. In talk therapy, witnesses provide verbal and nonverbal feedback about what they see and hear. The participant who has shared is validated and feels seen and heard. In drama therapy, participants receive validation through showing their story instead of just telling it. This allows them to literally be seen by others in the group in a three-dimensional way and be metaphorically acknowledged and accepted for their truth. A participant can even become his or her own witness. An example of this is when a participant tells a story, and the group acts it out, as in playback theatre. This allows the participant to step back and see the story from a distance. An additional aspect of witnessing happens during a drama therapy performance. The cast members in the show are witnesses to each other during rehearsal and performance. The audience, which is not part of the group, is invited in at the end to add their witnessing to the performance.

The Life-Drama Connection

The life-drama connection happens when participants are able to generalize the insights they have gained in drama therapy to their everyday lives. This can happen through a moment of insight during a scene or in the discussion that happens afterwards. One type of life-drama recognition is not better than the other. In any case, the life-drama connection must be made by participants through experience or reflection on their experience. Drama therapy allows participants to make discoveries as they become aware of their own actions. As anyone who has tried to tell someone else how to solve their problems knows, people tend not to remember what they are told when given advice or lectured; however, they do remember what they discover for themselves. That is when the lightbulb flashes on.

Transformation

Transformation is the goal of any therapeutic encounter, and in the best of all possible worlds, participants go through a series of transformations as therapy progresses. This goal relates closely to Yalom's therapeutic factor, catharsis. In most traditional therapies the participants verbalize their understanding of change; it is typically a cognitive experience. In drama therapy, participants get to engage and embody all the steps of the change: the mistakes, the missteps, the revisions, and the correct way of doing a task. Often transformation happens in incremental steps, which can be solidified in drama therapy through rehearsal and through watching the rehearsal of others. Sometimes change comes in a dramatic moment of insight that could be called *cathartic*. In addition, group creation of scenes, performances, and other dramatic enactments allows participants to develop, synthesize, and consolidate insights and new ways of being in the world throughout the process of working together.

The Drama Therapy Pie

Beginning students of drama therapy typically ask, "How can all these different methods and techniques be part of drama therapy? They are so different!" When Sally Bailey began teaching drama therapy at Kansas State University in 1999, she needed a way to clarify how all the disparate approaches of the drama therapy field fit together and relate to each other. To accomplish this, she created the drama therapy pie (see Figure 4).

Not every single intervention or approach of drama therapy is shown in this diagram. That would require so many slices of pie that the diagram would be impossible to read. As a result, the pie is drawn so the slices represent a few of the most well-known drama therapy approaches to provide a general idea of the range of interventions available.

Some of the interventions in the pie were modified from theatre techniques and shaped specifically to be used in drama therapy or psychodrama. For instance, DvT appears on its face to be pure improvisation, but it is not. DvT has been devised to contain unique structures like the witnessing circle. A DvT session does not move forward through the creation of individually improvised scenes; instead one improvisation flows into the next seamlessly without stopping and starting. In a sense, it is the dramatic form of word association. Some drama therapy interventions have not been changed from their original theatre form, but become therapy through their intentional focus to achieve therapeutic goals. A drama therapy group using devised theatre would focus on the treatment goals of the individual actors through the development and rehearsal of the play.

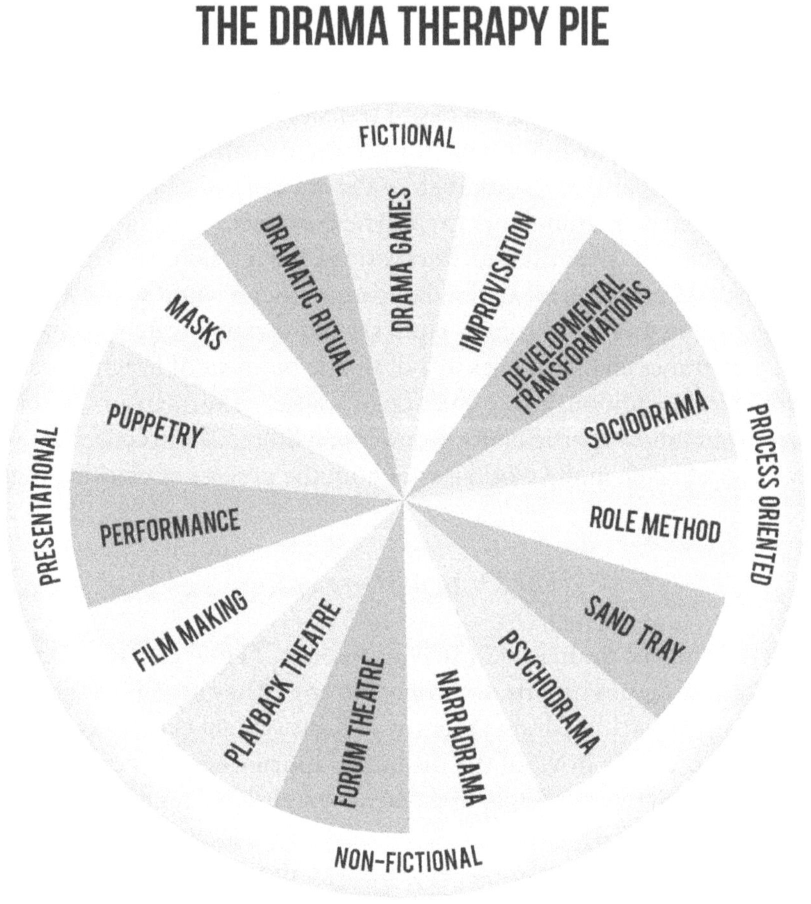

FIGURE 4: © Sally Bailey. 1999. Infographic Design © Sue Leo. 2019.

Also, the theme being developed would be relevant to the group's therapeutic goals as a whole. During rehearsals the drama therapist as director would keep in mind the therapeutic goals, strengths, and weaknesses of the actors in order to support and challenge their personal growth. While this sometimes happens in applied theatre or educational theatre, this kind of focus is not central; it is more often an unintended by-product.

There are two continuums represented on the drama therapy pie (see Figure 4). The slices on the upper half of the circle represent fictional interventions, and the slices on the bottom half represent nonfictional ones. For example, puppets are on the top because most puppets are fictional characters and are used to act out fictional scenarios. Psychodrama is at the bottom because the group spends most of its time acting out the actual story of the protagonist. The slices on the left half represent interventions that tend to be performance-oriented, and the slices on the right half represent ones that are more process-oriented (i.e., not done in front of an audience other than the drama therapy group). Playback theatre is on the left side of the pie because real stories of audience members are acted out by the playback troupe for the teller and the audience, while DvT is on the right side because whether it is done with individuals or a group, only the participants witness the work.

The continuums of the pie should not be seen as creating rigid placements for interventions. They are flexible guides to the way interventions tend to be used. The continuums reflect the fluid nature of many interventions, allowing the drama therapist to employ them for a variety of purposes. When using the pie and its continuums, think *and* rather than *either/or*. For example, an intervention, like playback theatre, that falls on the performance end of one continuum can be used as a process-oriented tool within a group to help participants learn how to listen to each other. Improvisation and role-play, which are placed toward the fictional end of the top-to-bottom continuum, can be focused on fictional or nonfictional material.

The drama therapy pie sits metaphorically on the plate of Renee Emunah's five phase integrative model because as the group progresses, different slices of the pie are used in different phases. The pie slices are not organized in a sequence that relate to the five phases. This is because with different diagnoses and individual needs, different interventions are appropriate in different phases. One of the purposes for this book is to explain how a drama therapist can choose appropriate interventions at different points in treatment in an ethical manner.

The Left to Right Continuum: Performance or Process-Oriented Interventions

One aspect of therapy that the drama therapy pie allows the therapist to consider is whether the participant would gain more insight from creating a presentational product (e.g., performance, puppet show, film, etc.) or from participating in process-oriented interventions that stay within the group. Preparing performances are usually more appropriate in later stages of group development. This in part is due to the need to create an ensemble before play creation or rehearsals begin. Ensemble-building would be phase one and two work. Rehearsal and performance would be in phase three and four. Phase five would involve deroling, talk-backs after the show, cast parties, and ending sessions for participants to discuss the insights gained and lessons learned. In individual therapy, the therapist and participant can consider using performance to create a self-revelatory performance or an autobiographical play in later phases, but first the therapeutic relationship needs to be developed.

Many process-oriented drama therapy interventions have inherent relationship-building components incorporated in phases one and two. For example, improvisation allows a back and forth interaction based on the improv rule *Yes, and* ... which requires that whatever "offer" one actor makes, the other must accept ("Yes,") and add on to ("and ..."):

A:	Would you like to go to the County Fair tonight?
B.	Yes, and we can buy some cotton candy.
A:	Yes, and I want to eat hot dogs, Boston baked beans, and Fried Twinkies.
A:	Yes, and we can go on the Ferris Wheel!
B:	Yes, and throw up all we've eaten when we reach the very top!

Yes, and ... allows participants to communicate more freely with each other, to develop trust with each other as they work together, and practice give-and-take. While an improvisation may be funny, the purpose of improvisation in drama therapy is not to entertain, but to build relationships, flexibility, spontaneity, and drama skills.

An intervention like playback theatre could be used as a process-oriented or a performance method. Learning playback forms needs to be done by the acting troupe in a rehearsal situation in order to prepare for a performance. However, sometimes a group is created only to play stories back to each other. In this case, the group would remain process-oriented. If the therapy group learned playback forms with the intention of performing for a public audience, the group would be performance-oriented. This application of playback has been used in schools where students who have been bullied are taught playback and then perform each other's stories to learn better how to deal with bullies.

The stakes rise when performance happens for the public. When performing playback, actors care about faithfully rendering the teller's story. The actors are witnessed by the audience as truth tellers, and this puts a great deal of pressure on them. Stresses on actors in a scripted play are different; they need to know their lines and blocking, entrances and exits. Even professional actors get stage fright, so the chances are that actors in a drama therapy group will too. Drama therapy participants will be better able to handle this kind of pressure in later phases of treatment.

Finally, rehearsals require the therapist and the group to put more focus on the creation of the play than on dealing with individual therapeutic issues. Once rehearsals start, the production train has left the station and is very difficult to stop! "The show must go on" is just the nature of the beast. Usually opening nights cannot be rescheduled. That does not mean interventions cannot be done, but the amount of time for therapeutic work must be limited if the play is going to be good enough for the participants to be successful. A therapist never wants to set their participants up for failure. If there are many emotional or behavioral issues that will interfere with rehearsals, perhaps the group is not ready to be working on a production.

The Top to Bottom Continuum: Fiction or Nonfiction

The top to bottom continuum of the drama therapy pie moves from fictional interventions at the top to nonfictional ones at the bottom. Fictional interventions like drama games and improvisation tend to have more distance than nonfictional ones like psychodrama or playback theatre. Starting with fictional interventions often helps participants engage in drama, because they are not so obviously revealing their personal vulnerability and secrets. This is why fiction is often used in phase one and two.

Picasso said, "We all know that Art is not truth. Art is a lie that makes us realize truth. ... The artist must know the manner whereby to convince others of the truthfulness of his lies" (Barr, 1980, p. 270). Because fiction can be seen as untrue rather than "a lie that reveals the truth," participants (and young therapists) might be tempted to jump into nonfiction work sooner than the group is ready. It is important that therapists take the time to prepare participants through the use of more distanced interventions and then bring in the life-drama connection in discussions after enactments. Having more distance in interventions early on allows participants time to feel comfortable doing drama and revealing personal information. Distance also allows them to identify dysfunctional life patterns through the lens of a metaphor or fairy tale. The dysfunction is not as threatening when it is distanced. Through fiction, it can be seen in its entirety, whereas in everyday life moments, participants may have little perspective on how they are entangled in their problems.

Fictional interventions can be useful as warm-ups to nonfictional interventions like psychodrama or forum theatre. Projective activities can be used by sociodrama groups to identify the shared social concern that the group will enact. Fictional patterns in devised plays allow a theme close to the participants' real lives to be explored without forcing anyone to self-disclose.

Using Both Continuums to Adjust Psychological Distance

Drama therapists must be aware of both continuums and how they affect each other. A group member entering the drama therapy group psychologically overdistanced, might need a less distanced drama therapy warm-up to create a state of balance or aesthetic distance. An improvisational warm-up playing with emotions like "emotional orchestra," "four corner dash," or "machines" may have enough aesthetic distance when applied to the group members to create balance. A participant, who begins to become psychologically underdistanced while acting in an improvisation, could be introduced to a puppet character, which provides more distance in the scene. Another way to balance an underdistanced participant might be to have them step out of the scene and become the director of it. This would require more cognitive processing and distance.

Some drama therapy interventions have built-in distancing devices. For instance, in psychodrama and sociodrama, the techniques of "walk and talk," "aside," "soliloquy," and "the magic screen," can give an underdistanced protagonist time to step out of a scene and verbalize thoughts and feelings. This adds more cognition into the actor's current mood and rearranges the balance between thought and feeling.

Conclusion

This chapter has focused on the underlying drama therapy principles that provide the foundation for the drama therapy decision tree. We have presented Susana Pendzik's metaphor of dramatic reality and Phil Jones's healing core elements of drama therapy, common to all drama therapy interventions. These are ingredients drama therapists consciously employ in their work.

Sally Bailey's drama therapy pie is a tool that creates a container for all the interventions that drama therapy has to offer. It allows drama therapists to evaluate if their interventions fall into a more traditional theatre approach (fiction/presentation), a more psychological approach (nonfiction/process) or another combination (fictional/process or nonfiction/presentation). This provides the participants with the right balance of aesthetic distance in order to reach insight and change (Bailey, 1999). In Chapter Three we will discuss diagnoses, classification systems, symptoms, and global treatment outcomes.

NOTE

1. *Narrative transportation* is the experience of being imaginatively transported into a book when reading or into a play or movie when watching. The body of the one transported stays in ordinary reality, but their imagination joins the characters of the book, play, or movie in a very real way (Greene & Carpenter, 2011). Being in dramatic reality means that the actor is not just imagining, but also fully embodying the character and story. See embodiment in Phil Jones's core concepts of drama therapy later in this chapter.

3

Foundations of Diagnoses and Global Functioning

This chapter discusses the tools used in treatment planning. The standard diagnostic protocols DSM-5 and ICD-11 are briefly reviewed, as they are the foundations on which clients are classified for treatment. Often the drama therapist comes into the equation after the diagnosis is made by a psychiatrist or psychologist and uses it to create a treatment plan. It is important to understand that treatment planning for a drama therapist comes from a strengths-based model, rather than a deficit-based one. This transforms the therapeutic approach from 'fixing' participants to 'empowering' them. In addition, there are two aspects of participant treatment that are important to review: the participants' symptoms and their global functioning.

DSM-5 and ICD-11[1]

The Diagnostic and Statistical Manual of Mental Disorders, Fifth Edition, DSM-5™ (2013), was revised by the American Psychiatric Association to improve communication between medical and mental health practitioners. The DSM-5 provides criteria and other pertinent information to aid practitioners in accurately diagnosing mental health disorders. It is often used to inform treatment decisions.

A diagnosis is the art of identifying which condition, disorder, or disease best explains a person's symptoms. The DSM-5 has been designed to dovetail with the ICD-11 (*International Classification of Diseases*), an international system of medical coding created by the World Health Organization (WHO) for documenting diagnoses, diseases, and symptoms as well as the social circumstances (Gaebel, 2015). ICD-11 was released on June 18, 2018, and can be accessed online (World Health Organization, 2018b). It was presented for endorsement at the 72nd World Health Assembly in May 2019. January 2022 is the date set for use of the new ICD-11 codes. For the purpose of this book, the DSM-5 and the ICD-11 will be discussed, as many drama therapists are required to use both coding systems for insurance billing and institutional documentation. While there is debate on whether a diagnosis is merely a construct or an actual disease (Greenberg, 2013), for the purpose of this book the two diagnostic systems are used to define and discuss a set of collective symptoms that a group of individuals share.

DSM-5

The DSM-5 is a categorical system, which lists the criteria for symptoms of mental disorders that are guidelines for making a diagnosis and informing clinical treatment. The DSM-5 defines a mental disorder as

> a syndrome characterized by clinically significant disturbance in an individual's cognition, emotion regulation, or behavior that reflects a dysfunction in the psychological, biological, or developmental processes underlying mental functioning. Mental disorders are usually associated with significant distress or disability in social, occupational, or other important activities. An expectable or culturally approved response to a common stressor or loss, such as the death of a loved one, is not a mental disorder. Socially deviant behavior (e.g., political, religious or sexual) and conflicts that are primarily between the individual and society are not mental disorders unless the deviance or conflict results from a dysfunction in the individual as described above.
>
> (American Psychiatric Association, 2013, p. 20)

In addition to the list of diagnostic criteria within each classification, there are features, which provide more details about additional considerations to assist in clarifying the disorder, such as diagnostic features, development and course of the disorder, and the risk and prognostic factors. 'Cultural Formation,' an independent section of the book, specifically addresses aspects of the cultural context of illness experience.

ICD-11

The ICD-11 is a broad diagnostic classification system, covering diseases, disorders, injuries, and other related health conditions. It is the international standard for reporting diseases and health conditions for all clinical and research purposes (World Health Organization, 2018a). The ICD-11 numerical codes are used by medical professionals the world over. Mental health clinicians in the United States are often required to use the ICD codes for billing insurance. The ICD-11 has narrative descriptions of disorders. Where there is the ability to quantify the criteria, the ICD-11 provides a measurable guideline to more clearly identify the criteria. The ICD-11 defines mental disorders this way:

> Mental, behavioural and neurodevelopmental disorders are syndromes characterized by clinically significant disturbance in an individual's cognition, emotional regulation or behaviour that reflects a dysfunction in the psychological, biological or developmental processes that underlie mental and behavioural functioning. These disturbances are usually associated with distress or impairment in personal, family, social, educational, occupational or other important areas of functioning.
>
> (World Health Organization, 2018c)

The DSM-5 and ICD-11: What Is the Difference?

Both DSM-5 and ICD-11 are examples of the medical model. An effort has been made to create more congruence between the DSM and the ICD in the most recent editions (American Psychiatric Association, 2013). The sections on mental, behavioral, and neurodevelopmental disorders in the ICD-11 are now hierarchically categorized in the same way as in the DSM-5. For each disorder the DSM-5 utilizes a list of criteria for diagnostic purposes, while the ICD-11 uses a narrative descriptive format. In addition, the ICD-11, when possible, gives quantifiable criteria for diagnosis, while the DSM-5 is more general.

The ICD-11 has excluded acute stress reaction and uncomplicated bereavement in the mental health section. Both of these diagnoses are addressed in ICD-11 in Section 24 "Factors Influencing Health Status or Contact with Health Services." Acute stress reaction is under the subsection "Problems Associated with Harmful and Traumatic Events." Uncomplicated bereavement is under the subsection "Problems Associated with Absence, Loss, or Death of Others." Moving these diagnoses out of the mental disorders category makes a statement that these conditions are not pathological, but do have the ability to impact an individual's overall health and functioning.

Sleep-wake disorders, sexual dysfunctions, and gender incongruence, included in the DSM-5, are not classified as mental, behavioral, or neurodevelopmental disorders in the ICD-11. These disorders are viewed purely from a medical perspective and are classified as medical conditions in sections 7 and 17, respectively. While they create physical, cognitive, and emotional functional impairments, the source of these impairments is considered to be a result of the reaction to a physiological illness, rather than being of a psychological origin.

Deficit-Based Versus Strength-Based Approaches

Many mental health clinicians struggle with the constraints of diagnostic classification systems and the pathologizing of clients that comes with labeling them with a diagnosis (Greenberg, 2013). However, insurance companies require the DSM or ICD for billing, and internationally scientists have agreed upon using DSM/ICD codes for research purposes. They create a common language researchers, mental health, and medical professionals use for communication. The difficulty many mental health clinicians have with the DSM and ICD is that they are deficit-based models.

Drama therapy comes from a strengths-based perspective, in part, because all the arts and creative arts therapies are strengths-based (Davidson, Shahar, Lawless, Sells, & Tondora, 2006; Hoffower, 2018; Lusseyran, 1994; Ornstein, 2006). Strengths-based approaches are part of the positive psychology movement, started by Martin E. P. Seligman (1991, 2002, 2011), Mihaly Csikszentmihalyi (1990, 1996), and Christopher Peterson (2006). Seligman (2002) identified three pillars of positive psychology: the study of positive emotions, positive traits (particularly strengths and virtues), and positive institutions. Strengths "are valued in almost every culture, valued in their own right, not just as a means to other ends, [and] they are malleable" (Seligman, 2002, p. 11). Being malleable means that strengths can be developed. According to Seligman,

> In comparing deficit-based and strengths-based approaches to therapy, Davidson et al. (2006) say, Mental health professionals are trained primarily to reduce or contain symptoms, ameliorate suffering, and perhaps, attempt to remediate dysfunction in our clients ... providers are active in identifying and addressing the intrusions and impacts of the illness while the person takes his or her medication as prescribed, follows the directives of others, and passively awaits improvement in his or her condition (with the possible exception of praying). Such a picture unfortunately leaves little room for a focus on facilitating the person's own efforts to establish, exercise, and eventually deploy an effective sense of social agency in doing battle with the illness.
>
> (2002, p. 159)

The strengths participants bring to therapy come from places of health and wellness that still reside within them, no matter how much despair, pain, or hopelessness they may be experiencing. As they work to express themselves through drama, movement, art, music, or writing, the healthy places begin to get stronger and respond to the freedom for self-expression and control that the arts provide (Davidson et al., 2006; Hoffower, 2018; Van Lith, Fenner, & Schofield, 2010). Beginning with self-expression, participants quickly move to connection, communication, and meaning-making. Hope begins to develop out of their hopelessness and their locus of control (LOC) slowly becomes more internal as their motivation to reengage in life grows (Davidson et al., 2006; Heise, 2014; Spandler, Secker, Kent, Hacking, & Shenton, 2007).

Making "good," "aesthetic," or "pleasing" art is not the focus of the creative arts therapies; instead the goal is self-expression, self-exploration, and meaning-making. A positive offshoot of these actions is that participants begin to see themselves as whole individuals, not stigmatized invalids:

> [A]bove and beyond being seen as someone with some artistic ability ... the production of artwork enabled [our clients] to develop or consolidate a renewed identity in the world, challenging their identity as being primarily defined by their mental ill-health.
>
> (Spandler et al., 2007, pp. 795–796)

Another aspect of the strengths-based approach of the creative arts therapies is that play, an aspect of all the arts, is incorporated, and play is fun. Because work done through the deficit-based model focuses on what is wrong, therapy can be painful. In describing the results of an arts-based, experiential group for children in foster care, Diana Coholic and her coresearchers (2012) remarked that:

> Indeed, it was through the experience of fun that some of the children developed emotional regulation, which enabled more effective coping with a variety of challenges and that some improved their self-awareness and felt better about themselves. ... The experience of fun should not be divorced from learning new skills and awareness. ... It is fun that keeps the child emotionally receptive so that the intense positive messages can slip through her defenses.
>
> (p. 354)

On the face of it, the notion of pairing a deficit-based diagnostic system with strength-based treatment planning may seem paradoxical. However, drama therapy is strong enough to hold the paradox, as it engages participants through play and imagination. Drama therapy treatment interventions follow the improvisation rule of "Yes, and ..." instead of "No" or "Maybe, but ..." When engaged in drama therapy, participants' strengths are incorporated to develop those strengths and heal their deficits.

Having fun is another reason why phase one involves dramatic play; players are enticed to engage. A recovering addict from a Second Genesis drama therapy group wrote a letter about what drama therapy meant to him. He said:

> I have found out a lot about my real self—who I am, what I am, my likes and dislikes, and how I react to things, feelings, and emotions. Part of what taught me this new way of life were the things I learned in drama therapy. It renewed the child in me. It gave me happiness inside—something I had lost. So much an addict needs self-esteem. Drama helped me develop it. Trust, love, and caring are other qualities that I learned about through drama. Drama showed me how to interact with others. Most of all, it gave me a way to have excitement in my life without the use of drugs. I can have fun being me without having to put on a mask.
>
> (personal communication, 1993)

The embodiment and action focus of drama therapy draws on participants' strengths. In order to move into action, participants need to want to get up and connect. A drama game is motivating because it feels good physically. Insight can be discovered through one's own body, instead of from a lecture. For example, the drama game "machines" can improve emotional regulation (ER). Each person uses a movement and a sound to connect to and become part of a real or imaginary machine. After the machine is created, the therapist can slow down or speed up the machine, helping group members create an awareness of their physiology. The players are initially focused on engaging with each other and being silly. After players experience the speed changes, the therapist can ask, "OK, now what was the difference between moving quickly and moving slowly?" The reflections that result lead them to develop a new self-awareness, which leads to new skills, such as understanding body boundaries and self-control. A variation called "emotion machines" releases pent-up emotions. In this game all sounds and motions must express one identified emotion. Participants realize that they can change how they feel through physical action that releases uncomfortable emotions and enhances enjoyable ones.

Regardless of whether deficit- or strengths-based orientations are used, diagnoses are usually the springboard into a treatment plan. Drama therapists are very good at making lemonade out of lemons. They can start with a deficit-based diagnosis and flip the approach to be strengths-based. Being able to speak DSM/ICD allows drama therapists to have a common language with other therapists on treatment teams and other medical and mental health professionals working across the health-care fields while still accentuating the positive in terms of treatment interventions.

Symptoms Versus Global Functioning

In creating treatment goals and objectives, there are two elements of participant functioning within any diagnosis to grapple with. One is to deal with the symptoms. Symptoms for a participant with autism spectrum disorder (ASD) probably include communication problems, ritualistic behaviors, and low affect. Any or all of them could become the focus of a drama therapy intervention. The other components of a diagnosis are the global areas of functioning. An individual with ASD might experience global functioning problems in executive functioning (EF), sensory integration (SI), and flexibility. These global areas cross diagnostic categories. Global areas of functioning are often ignored in the symptom criteria of diagnoses, because they do not help the clinician differentiate between multiple diagnoses. The symptoms of the diagnosis often drive the decisions about treatment planning. It is easier to operationally define symptoms than to define global functioning. However, global functioning areas can impact behavior change as well.

Drama therapy is so effective because drama therapy interventions often target global functioning at the same time as symptoms. It is important for early career drama therapists to understand global functioning because insurance companies often recognize global functioning outcomes equally with symptom outcomes. In the remaining part of the chapter, the following aspects of global functioning will be addressed: creativity, SI, EF, empathy, and LOC.

Creativity contributes to the development of spontaneity and flexibility. These three psychological competencies work together to increase problem-solving abilities, meaning making, setting and achieving goals, and finding satisfaction in life. People who are creative tend to develop self-confidence and belief in themselves. Their creative endeavors are proof that they can succeed.

SI, EF, and empathy are processes that are part of the neurological and physiological systems. Deficits show up within these systems in a variety of mental health diagnoses. These deficits can be successfully addressed through drama therapy. It makes sense to talk about them here as contained units, rather than address them within each diagnosis. The development of empathy is a need for many participants who have DSM diagnoses. Lack of empathy for some participants result from dysfunctions created by social disconnection and social media or due to trauma and family disruption.

Finally, LOC may be one of the core aspects of global functioning that drama therapy inherently modifies. One of the main purposes of therapy in an individualistic culture is to empower the participant to function independently in a healthy manner. Feeling empowered and acting independently indicate a movement from external to internal LOC. Drama therapy is ideal for increasing internal LOC because of the many opportunities participants have to engage in action and effect change on self and others in the group. Metaphorically, participants are able to make choices and take control of their lives in dramatic enactments, scripted or improvisational. The insights gained from these experiences can be generalized into everyday life.

Creativity

Creativity is one of those concepts that has no single operational definition. Sawyer (2006) says that creativity is not a scientific concept, but a "culturally and historically specific idea that changes from one country to another and from one century to another" (p. 36). A creative process or product is both novel and appropriate (i.e., socially valuable to the community in which one lives). In other words, each culture decides what is creative based on its values, needs, and history. Creativity is related to specific domains: physics, poetry, theatre, and so on. The experts within the specific domain get to decide whether something new is creative (Sawyer, 2006).

Creativity and spontaneity are basic to any art modality, especially drama therapy as it relies on so many aspects of improvisational drama. Jacob Moreno, the founder of psychodrama, sociodrama, and sociometry, placed creativity and spontaneity as central aspects of his methods (Kipper, Davelaar, & Herst, 2009; Moreno, 1987, 1993). Creativity has been linked to important positive outcomes, such as increased problem-solving, critical thinking, and divergent thinking, and decreases in stress, anxiety, and mood disturbances (Sowden, Clements, Redlich, & Lewis, 2015; Stuckey & Nobel, 2010).

> When people are invited to work with creative and artistic processes that affect more than their identity with illness, they are more able to "create congruence between their affective states and their conceptual sense making."
>
> (Yorks & Kasl as cited in Stuckey & Nobel, 2010, p. 261)

The Creative Process

The creative process is divided into steps that are very similar to the steps of problem-solving: *preparation, incubation, insight,* and *verification.* Verification consists of two steps: *evaluation* and *elaboration* (Sawyer, 2006). Because creativity is such an important process of drama therapy, details of these steps follow.

Preparation
When a problem presents itself, the creator enters a preparation period. Preparation consists of all the knowledge previously gathered by the creator in the domain in which the problem exists, and all the specific research the creator is doing currently on the problem. Any conscious consideration and deliberation on the problem is considered part of preparation.

Incubation
Incubation is when the information gathered "percolates" in the unconscious mind of the creative person. Sometimes the percolation happens partly during the preparation; sometimes all of it comes after preparation. No one is exactly sure what happens during incubation, because so much of it is done below the level of awareness, but the best guess is that the gathered information is pulled apart into smaller components and reassembled into a new idea.

Insight
Insight is that "Aha!" moment of recognition when a new idea appears in consciousness to solve the problem. Therapy is a process in which participants seek insights on their behavior, so it bears spending a few paragraphs exploring exactly where insights come from and how a therapist can help participants generate them. Gary Klein (2013), an organizational psychologist, has explored how insights happen. He says:

> An insight is a leap, an unpredictable leap, to a related but different story [from the story a person has been telling him/herself]. It catches us by surprise because it isn't the product of conscious, deliberate, deductive, or statistical inference ... The insight usually arrives as a coherent new story.
>
> (p. 245)

Verification
Finally, the creative idea is verified. In this final stage, the person evaluates the idea. A good idea needs to be novel and appropriate to solve the problem. Then the idea must be elaborated on. That is often when the real work begins: converting the new idea into a finished product. The product could be a fully articulated theory, a machine, a book, a song, a painting, or an improvised scene (Sawyer, 2006).

Big C *and Little* c *Creativity*

Creativity comes in two types: Big C and little *c*. Creativity with a big C is when artists and inventors create new work that change our ideas and behaviors within or across cultures. Creativity with a little *c* is whenever a person solves an everyday problem in an original way. Everyone has the potential to develop their creativity in different domains; however, not everyone has access to the resources, training, social support, or time to develop their innate creativity in big *C* areas (Sawyer, 2006). Drama therapists are focused on the expansion of the little *c* in participants.

Sawyer (2006), who has spent most of his psychology career studying creativity, lists the following aspects of little *c* everyday creativity in a group: collaborative, improvised, emerges unpredictably from a group of people, and depends on shared cultural knowledge. In everyday creativity, the process is the product, and the focus is about social encounters. If these are the challenges of everyday life, which we are all called upon to solve, then clearly drama therapy provides many opportunities to practice and grow one's little *c* creativity skills.

Most often drama therapy creativity is a group creative process. This provides participants with practice in brainstorming, respecting and accepting others' ideas, interacting, sharing the building of a scene with others, and making a compromise when another's idea might solve a problem better than one's own idea. Participants can engage in a short creative process (an improvised scene or a theatre game) or a longer, more elaborate creative product (writing and mounting a theatrical production).

Improvisation is one of the major tools involved in the preparation and elaboration stages of the creative process. Experience in improvising is useful because most aspects of life are improvisational. Even everyday conversations are created on the fly. Improvisation incorporates conscious and unconscious processes. Practicing improvisation in a drama therapy group develops these skills that can later be generalized to life (an instance of the life-drama connection). Consciously, the actor must pay attention to what the other actors are saying and respond appropriately to them with a new line that moves the scene forward.

If one actor said, "At the store we need to get bread, milk, and eggs ..." It would be inappropriate for the other actor to respond with, "I agree, going to the hospital is the best way to deal with this emergency." Even if it were a comic improv, the two actors are not talking *with* each other. Consciously and unconsciously, the actors respond to the offer made by the other actor, trying to generate an appropriate, but novel response that will move the scene forward and develop both of their characters. Focus and concentration are involved, as well as flexibly switching attention back and forth between conscious and unconscious processing. The icing on the cake is that the actors have the joyful experience of practicing the creative process: creating the characters, dialogue, and story of a scene out of their imaginations. That experience teaches how the whole creative process is completed.

In addition to creative group work, each insight a participant has as the result of a drama therapy intervention is a creative act. When a variety of information learned about the self comes together in a new way with functioning more appropriately in the world, the participant has an "Aha!" experience. Sometimes personal insights arise during the creation of a scene. Sometimes it arises afterwards during the group discussion. For example, a participant realizes that he has few friends and no romantic partners because of habitually blocking the offers of others.

Can all participants engage in the creative process? Yes. Psychologists have found evidence that creativity is not tied to intelligence (Sawyer, 2006). The mental processes that are involved in creativity are basic ones typically used by all. The "magic tube," a creativity game, can be played with everyone from gifted adolescents to very low functioning individuals with intellectual and developmental disabilities and from young children to older adults. In this game a paper towel tube is passed around the circle, and each person uses it to demonstrate a different object it could be. Because it is based on a concrete, seeable, touchable object, the "magic tube" can be used as a tool to teach participants, who have difficulty with abstract thinking, how to use their imagination, create metaphors, and think more symbolically.

Spontaneity

Spontaneity is a necessary ingredient for creativity. Some people mistakenly think creativity and spontaneity are the same, but they are not. Moreno (1993) believed that spontaneity is a psychological energy of short duration which serves as the catalyst for creativity. Spontaneity only exists in the here and now, which makes it a perfect resource for engaging participants in a creative form of therapy. It sparks connection to the moment and the exploration at hand, motivating curiosity and freeing participants from inhibitions and shyness, which might hold them back.

Unfortunately, spontaneity is sometimes misinterpreted as being wildly uninhibited and inappropriate. This is not how the term spontaneity is intended to be used in terms of creativity. In describing spontaneity, Moreno (1987) says,

> The term "spontaneous" is often used to describe subjects whose control of their actions is diminished .... Disorderly conduct and emotionalism resulting from impulsive action are far from being desiderata of spontaneity work. Instead, they belong more in the realm of the pathology of spontaneity.
>
> (pp. 42–43)

Research positively correlates spontaneity to "well-being, self-efficacy, and self-esteem and negatively correlate[s] it to anxiety, stress, and obsessive-compulsive tendencies" (Kipper et al., 2009, p. 330). Furthermore, individuals who are inhibited as opposed to spontaneous are "characterized by reduced expressiveness, unemotional language, and shyness" (Kipper et al., 2009, p. 332). Results from a pair of experiments evaluating spontaneity in college students conducted by Kipper and colleagues (2009) showed that "the greater spontaneity the lower the maladaptive inhibition" (p. 333).

Kipper compares spontaneity and the experiential state of mind it creates to the *flow experience* (Csikszentmihalyi, 1990, 1996), an optimal state where the sense of time disappears, the task feels effortless and automatic, and the person focuses only on the action being engaged in. Typically, flow is created only when the difficulty of the task is just beyond the ability level of the person. If the task is too easy or too hard, flow is not experienced. Improvisation is the perfect task to generate feelings of flow, especially if the drama therapist has set up the scene in a way that adapts the rules and guidelines for the scene to the abilities of the participants.

Inability to be spontaneous can create major blocks in functionality. Some participants diagnosed with autism spectrum disorder (ASD) experience rigidity in their thoughts and behavior. In order to control their world, they will not try unfamiliar activities. They have difficulty making decisions and taking risks; they need to think about what to do for so long that the rest of the group can become bored or frustrated waiting for them. To train participants like this in spontaneity, it is important to start small and create realistic choices, so the activity becomes a game that relates to real life. For instance, instead of playing a game where players pantomime a magical creature, adapt the game so players pantomime real-life professions. Build slowly from there by adding the acting out of more imaginary creatures in a later replaying of the game. If the participants have learned to be spontaneous in one area, like playing video games, try explaining spontaneity by saying, "It's like when you are playing video games, and you have to react quickly, or you lose the battle and have to start the game over."

Certain participants, for instance, people who have bipolar disorder, borderline personality disorder, or attention deficit hyperactivity disorder (ADHD), can be too spontaneous. The drama therapist may need to explain that there are boundaries to spontaneity, and those boundaries have to do with following the rules and respecting safety within the group. Pit the players' investment in the project or their enjoyment of the dramatic play against their impulsivity to break the rules.

Flexibility

Flexibility is connected to spontaneity. It is a willingness to explore other possible beliefs than what was previously believed, or other ways of doing things than what was previously done. To be willing to be flexible means being willing to be vulnerable and take a risk and fail. Most beginners in Western cultures are not accustomed to being vulnerable or failing. Participants who are beginning therapy are even less so, as they are most likely facing a lot of failure due to their current problems.

Developing flexibility is important to living a healthy life, because one needs to be willing to try new solutions when the old ones do not work. Improvisation is a fun way to begin learning those skills. There is even an improv game in which mistakes are made on purpose, and players are applauded for it. In another improv game, everyone must tell a story about when they failed or did something stupid, and when each story is finished, the whole group cheers and celebrates the failure.

Sensory Integration

Sensory integration (SI) is the ability to take in, combine, and comprehend all the messages from the senses that are constantly bombarding the brain. The sensory system includes vision, hearing, smell, taste, touch, balance, proprioception, and interoception. *Proprioception* is the sense of how the body is positioned in space in relation to the world. *Interoception* includes pressure, pain, heat, cold, hunger, thirst, and other interior perceptions in the viscera or organs of the body (Ceunen, Vlaeyen, & Van Diest, 2016). When the senses are well integrated, it is as if there is a soundboard with volume control and a mixer in the brain that balances and adjusts the incoming messages of the senses. Sensory input can be adjusted up or down, allowing the person to focus on certain messages and ignore others by muting them. In this way, we are able to pay close attention to one particular sense or environmental aspect, while blocking out others. For instance, students sitting in a classroom need to be able to focus on what the teacher is saying rather than be distracted by the lawn mower cutting the grass outside.

Disordered SI can be an issue in ASD, learning disabilities, ADHD, post-traumatic stress disorder (PTSD), and schizophrenia. To deal with SI problems, accommodations can be made in the drama therapy space to lower distractions and unpleasant sensory experiences. Accommodations can also be made in the choice of interventions. Warm-up games with constantly changing movements and noises that are passed around the circle in irregular patterns will overload participants' integration abilities. Instead plan simple go-around games where each person in the circle takes a turn to pass the face or act out their favorite animal. If players are not ready to be put on the spot to pantomime or respond solo, there are games that require unison work or small group interactions. Certain awareness activities can help participants focus on just one sense at a time: identifying sounds coming from different locations in the room or changing one thing about their appearance and having a partner guess what is different. Games with more complexity or speed can be added slowly as participants develop trust, group cohesion, and comfort with activities.

Executive Functioning

Executive functioning (EF) are processes involved in neurological and physiological systems. Deficits show up within these systems in a variety of mental health diagnoses. All of these deficits can be successfully addressed through drama therapy. It makes sense to talk about them here as contained units. Metacognition, one aspect of EF, needs to be mentioned in particular because there is often a misunderstanding on the part of non-drama therapists that drama therapy consists only of doing and not of reflecting on what was done. Metacognition is part of all therapeutic endeavors, as psychological change involves becoming more aware of one's self in relation to one's inner being and the surrounding world. Emotional and behavior regulation, also aspects of EF, are involved in initiating appropriate and inhibiting inappropriate emotions and behaviors.

Executive Functioning is an "umbrella construct for a collection of interrelated functions" located in the prefrontal lobes of the brain (Gioia, Isquith, Retzlaff, & Espy, 2002, p. 250). Unfortunately, EF is another one of those constructs that everyone defines a little bit differently. As recently as 2014, Najdowski, Persicke, and Kung stated, "The term executive function refers to the hypothesized brain processes that control other brain processes. Most researchers agree that the term is exceedingly broad, and there is little consensus on the definition" (p. 355). In a nutshell, EF are those mental processes that allow us to achieve goals and manage life tasks. Elkhonon Goldberg (2009) says that the "[f]rontal lobes are critical for every successful learning process, for motivation and attention," (p. 5) and that EF are "to the brain what a conductor is to an orchestra, a general is to an army, the chief executive officer is to a corporation" (p. 4). Examples of EF include the ability to focus, plan, make decisions, shift attention between tasks, and the emotional and behavioral aspects of self-control.

For the purposes of this book, the authors have made an executive decision about how we are going to organize our discussion of EF. We are saying that there are three major dimensional constructs of EF: metacognition (thoughts), emotional regulation (ER, feelings), and behavioral regulation (BR, actions). There are skills that fit within the boundaries of one construct or work in coexistence with two or three: working memory, attention, shifting attention, sequencing, shifting emotions, self-reflection, initiation, inhibition, task planning and organization, and task monitoring. Since many of these components cross more than one EF construct, we will talk about each of them as separate entities so as not to confuse the reader.

Metacognition

Metacognition is the awareness of and ability to evaluate one's own thought process. In other words, it is thinking about thinking. This can be what one knows about cognition in general or about one's own cognition (Schraw & Moshman, 1995). In terms of EF, planning, task organization, task monitoring and evaluation, and self-reflection are considered a part of metacognition. However, we will describe these separately from metacognition because in designing treatment plans, the larger concept of metacognition can be a treatment goal, but the components are more appropriate for treatment objectives (more on treatment planning in the following chapter).

For participants to be able to understand themselves, they have to be able to recognize their thoughts and feelings. They also have to be able to understand how those thoughts and feelings relate to their personality, sense of self, and past experience. They must be able to connect how those thoughts and feelings are driving their current behavior. They need to develop what Grant (2001) calls psychological mindedness and learn the way their mind works: in short, come to understand their own psychology.

In order to think about your thoughts, you have to access them and then monitor them: attune to, pay attention to, and remember them (Baker & Brown, 1984; National Research Council, 2000). There are very specific strategies that drama therapy naturally incorporates which help develop metacognition. As participants succeed at drama therapy interventions, they are guided by the drama therapist through group discussions to understand their strengths and weaknesses, recognize their limits, and accept the possibility that they can surpass what they have seen as their limits.

The biggest obstacle to metacognition is the amount of intellectual effort that it requires; especially for someone who does not regularly do it. Participants sense the difficulty of the process and that is often why they avoid therapy. Drama therapy is sneaky about this and can lure participants into being curious about their thought processes. Participants find themselves in the middle of the therapeutic process before they realize it. They end up becoming curious about what happened in the intervention they just did, and this encourages metacognition.

Drama therapy encourages active cognition during and after interventions. When the drama therapist begins group discussions with open-ended questions, participants learn how to listen to and ask themselves questions. Later that will translate into the ability to monitor self-talk to see if what they are saying to themselves internally is helping or hindering them. This type of internal skill-building moves participants from being cognitively passive to being cognitively active.

Working Memory

Working memory holds information in consciousness where goals are created, plans are made, and problems are solved. Daniel Siegel (1999) calls it *the chalkboard of the mind*. Information from long-term memory is pulled to the frontal lobes where it can be mixed with new information needed for completing a task. Goldberg (2009) defines this action as "the selection of task-relevant information" (p. 94). No one knows exactly how information is manipulated once it is in working memory; many of its processes are still a mystery.

Long-term, short-term, and working memory can be confusing terms. *Long-term memory* is where information is stored for extended periods of time in the brain. Facts are stored in long-term memory as declarative memories. Stories about our personal experiences are in long-term memory as part of *episodic memory*. Information about how to do actions like drive a car or ride a bike are stored as *procedural memory*. Exactly where long-term memory is located in the brain is not known. Scientists currently believe parts of a memory are stored in different places in the brain and then pulled together when brought into consciousness in working memory (Corkin, 2013; Cowan, 2008).

When we receive new information, it is held first in short-term memory. This is transferred to working memory, and then to long-term memory, or it is forgotten. The term *working memory* has not always been seen as distinct from short-term memory (Cowan, 2008). Memory researchers consider *short-term memory* as a mental process that deals with information in the immediate present. Items in short term memory tend to last no more than 30 seconds, unless it is sent to working memory where it can be rehearsed or manipulated (Corkin, 2013). Working memory uses information from short-term memory and long-term memory. As its name suggests, working memory manipulates that information for a cognitive purpose. In a sense, it is a blank slate or clipboard to which information can be sent and rearranged.

At one point neuroscientists (Miller, Galanter, & Pribram, 1960) believed that most people could hold up to seven chunks of information in their working memory (plus or minus two chunks), but currently the belief is that the average number of chunks is closer to four plus-or-minus two chunks (Stein, 2007). Individuals who have attention deficits or emotional overloads involved in their diagnosis are able to hold fewer items than the average. This means that, depending on one's physical or mental health, working memory can expand or contract to a degree. A participant with anxiety who is overloaded with fearful ruminations or a recent widow overwhelmed by grief will both have difficulty comprehending their boss's directions about how to do a job. If their doctor gives them instructions on how to take medication, they might not retain it. Knowing this can help the therapist communicate better. First, capture the participant's attention, then slowly, deliberately, make sure the message is heard. Multiple ways of delivering information may be helpful: spoken, written, and pictorial.

Information can be manipulated in the working memory in verbal or visuospatial form (Goldberg, 2009). Visuospatial information provides more complex information than words because an image can combine many pieces of data together. So there *is* truth to the saying, "A picture is worth a thousand words."

Because of the limited number of chunks of information that can be held at one time, items do not stay in working memory long. If the person is to continue deliberating about the same information, a great deal of attention and effort must be brought to bear so it is not forgotten (Goldberg, 2009). As soon as a different fact, image, or distraction is brought in, one, two, or all of the items that were being held will vanish. If one wants to continue thinking about the same items, they have to be retrieved again from long-term memory.

"Change three" is a drama game that can motivate participants who have smaller capacities in their working memory to exercise and expand their volume. Group members are challenged to remember as much as they can about one player's appearance. That player will go somewhere they cannot be seen and will change three things about their appearance. Because no one knows what will be removed, added, or changed, group members need to hold as many aspects of the changer's appearance in their working memory.

Many theatre games enhance working memory partly because they are embodied. Researchers have looked at movement, body gestures, and working memory. Schaefer (2018) did a study to determine if physical movement related to a cognitive task would enhance memory. She tested participants in two conditions: some performed the task while standing still and some performed it in the embodied condition. Participants in the embodied condition remembered more.

Attention

Attention is comprised of two components: attenuation and sustaining focus. *Attenuation* involves choosing where to focus your awareness. You could attenuate to a teacher's lecture or to your iPhone. Making that choice is called *selective attention*. However, the ability to attenuate can fail. Failure can be internal or external. An *internal failure* is when the skill to attenuate is missing, or the capacity to attenuate is diminished. This would be the case for someone who had a cognitive delay or severe ADHD. *External failure* relates to the stimuli not being strong enough to capture your attention. An external failure might occur if you are trying to read a book, but are distracted by very loud music coming from the next room.

The second component of attention is *sustaining focus* on the object to which you have attenuated. Failure to sustain focus can be due to a lack of skill or the strength of a distraction. When dealing with attention issues, assessing whether the root cause is failure to attenuate or sustain focus can be difficult. This can be controlled for and assessed in laboratory situations, but not always in real life.

Attention is necessary in order to focus on tasks in working memory or in physical action. Cognitive disorders like ADHD may limit attention spans, making it difficult for a person to stay with a thought, activity, or goal. Likewise, mental illnesses like depression or medications for a condition may interfere with the functioning of attention, making it difficult to focus clearly and stay focused.

A game that deals with attenuation is "zip-zap-zop." Players must attenuate each time someone in the circle passes them a zip, a zap, or a zop. This game moves quickly, and no one knows when or where a zip, zap, or zop will come from or go to. This works as an excellent warm-up and energizer game for the same reason as it works on attenuation: it encourages alertness in players.

A drama game that addresses both attenuation and sustaining focus is "mirroring." One partner moves slowly and the other copies the first for a series of slow, deliberate, extended motions. The initial moment of paying attention to the leading partner involves attenuation by the mirroring partner, and following the leading partner requires sustaining focus.

Shifting Attention

Shifting attention involves the ability to shift from one object of focus to another. This is a different skill-set from focusing attention. To shift attention, you have to be able to attenuate to something new while simultaneously choosing not to focus on the previous stimuli. The rapidity at which shifting attention can be done makes it appear as if one is paying attention to two things at once, but researchers have discovered that this is not possible (Ophir, Nass, & Wagner, 2009).

The failure to shift attention can be caused by an internal or external failure. An example of an internal failure could be caused by obsessive compulsive disorder (OCD), which involves having difficulty in disengaging attention from certain thoughts or actions. An external failure would relate to the strength of the competing stimuli. For example, students are often so engaged with their electronic devices that the professor could be standing on her head, and they still would not look up.

"Pass the sound, pass the movement" involves passing a sound and a movement from player to player around a circle. When a player accepts the sound and movement, attention shifts to the player on the right and then the player must shift attention to the player on the left in order to pass it. This appears to be simple, especially in the version of the game when the sound and movement does not change, but as layers of complexity are added, more concentration is needed for the shift to happen smoothly.

Another game that many group members enjoy is the "night at the museum" (also known as "museum guard"). This game involves the majority of the group focusing on the task of stealing keys from the museum guard. They pretend to be statues that come to life and must sneak up on the guard, steal the keys, and sneak out of the museum without being caught. In order to do this successfully, attention needs to shift between the guard, the keys, and other members of the group as they work together to trick the guard.

Sequencing

Sequencing is the ability to arrange and remember language, thoughts, information, and actions in an order that is useful or makes sense. The alphabet has a given sequence, as does any task. Some sequences are arbitrary (the alphabet), others are logical (a mathematical proof), and some are based in natural processes (growth and development). Sequencing can also be based on time (first, second, third or beginning, middle, end). Some types of sequencing involve cause and effect: one action produces a consequence.

Most tasks can be broken down into a series of subtasks. To complete the task, the sequence of the subtasks must be accomplished in order. For instance, if you want to seal a letter into an envelope, start by folding the letter in thirds, then insert it into the envelope, then run your tongue across the glue on the flap of the envelope, then put the envelope down on the table and seal the flap by pressing it down. If you forget the sequence of the subtasks, you might seal the envelope before the letter is inside. Without the ability to sequence, no problem could be solved, no book could be read, no meals could be cooked. In fact, our whole day is based on the ability to sequence.

A participant who has difficulty with sequencing might have difficulty following directions. A useful way to handle this is to give one instruction at a time. For example, for a name game, first say, "Everyone stand in a circle." Wait until everyone is in the circle. Then say, "Everyone think of a different movement that shows something you like to do." Wait for everyone to think of something. "Are you ready? Great! Let's go around the circle, and each person show your movement and say your name."

Playwriting involves sequencing. The action of any scene develops in a specific pattern following the Fedder's Four sequence: I want … But … However … So (as cited in Bailey, 2009). Each scene builds on the one before it from the opening scene to the climax and the completion of the conflict (denouement).

"Pattern ball passing" requires players to remember several different sequences as one to four balls are passed around a circle in specific patterns. The player must remember that the blue ball from Phil must be passed to Jill while the red ball from Fred must be passed to Quincy. When the players synchronize the ball passing effectively, the rhythm supports the remembering of the sequence.

Emotional Regulation

Emotional regulation (ER) is the ability to control one's emotions. ER involves thoughts, feelings, behaviors, and physiological responses that act upon each other. ER requires two steps. First, one must recognize the emotion by becoming aware of the cognitive, physiological, and behavioral responses to a stimulus. The second step relates to the expression of the emotion. Emotions are fundamentally embodied (Niedenthal, 2007), so typically, as they are experienced, they will also be expressed physically and behaviorally. For example, when a person feels adrenaline rushing through their body, sees red, feels their face flushing, notices both their hands are clenched, and thinks, "I want to hit him," that person is most likely angry. If the emotion has not yet been expressed, the person must decide as part of ER whether or not to express it.

Emotion is displayed at a particular intensity. If a person has ER, it is possible to choose the intensity and manner in which the emotion is displayed. This means the person has the ability to increase, decrease, or maintain the emotion. It also can mean transitioning from one emotion to a different one, when appropriate. Upon becoming angry, someone with strong ER might take a deep breath, count to ten, and then engage in a civil conversation about the problem, while someone with poor ER might become enraged and begin screaming.

Emotional Regulation skills must be learned. ER typically develops with age; however, many participants in therapy need to develop these skills. Drama therapy can be used to build them.

When an emotion is not displayed, it is important to understand if the lack of expression is because: the individual is able to recognize the emotion, but consciously chooses not to express it; is unable to recognize the emotion; or is unaware because of an unconscious defense mechanism, such as repression. Making a conscious choice not to express an emotion is a type of ER, while repression or inability to recognize emotion are types of emotional dysregulation.

The inability to recognize an emotion could be due to alexithymia, as when a traumatized person feels numb. If the person is feeling emotionally flooded, it is possible that specific emotions cannot be distinguished from the physical experience of feeling overwhelmed. This happens when a participant experiences a rush of adrenalin and is unable to interpret whether the rush is being caused by excitement, fear, or anger. Regardless of the reason, if the emotion is not identified, ER cannot occur.

Research has shown that targeted attention and knowledge strategies are better ER mechanisms than venting emotions through bodily expressions (Gross, 1998). Drama therapy involves many interventions that allow emotional expression and regulation skills to be learned and practiced. Through creating characters in improvisations, participants learn how to control the intensity of the emotions they are expressing. They come to understand that the emotion belongs to the character they are playing. This creates a distance from the emotion, allowing participants to experiment with experiencing it, escalating it, de-escalating it, and letting it transform into another emotion. For instance, if a participant is playing an angry customer in an improvisation, the anger being expressed has to be believable or the other actors will be unable to respond appropriately. The actor learns that the character is angry; the actor is not. Through practice, the actor learns to separate from the emotion through the dual consciousness created when functioning simultaneously as actor and character (Emunah, 2020). If by chance the actor is still feeling the emotion when the scene is over, deroling will allow the anger to be let go, helping the actor separate from the character (Bailey & Dickinson, 2016). In essence, through enroling and deroling, participants learn how to express and modulate emotion.

A drama game called "emotion thermometer" can assist participants to understand how to regulate the intensity of their emotions. As participants respond to instructions to increase or decrease the intensity of an embodied emotion, they realize that they can control how the emotion is expressed and changed. An "emotion spectrogram" and "emotion sculpting" are other interventions that help participants practice aspects of emotions.

Behavioral Regulation

Behavioral Regulation involves the choice of inhibiting or expressing actions related to emotional stimuli, thoughts, or environmental cues. Similar to ER, BR is not just the choice of whether to express an action or not; it also involves action management related to choosing the appropriate action and intensity of that action. For instance, if your boss makes a condescending remark, you could ignore the comment, stride out of the room and slam the door, or confront the behavior in a civil manner ("When you say that to me, I feel ...").

The ability to regulate behavior is often judged by social norms and rules. Within certain cultures it is acceptable to complain vociferously about a problem. In other cultures, complaining is seen as an inability to regulate emotions or deal head-on with a problem. Likewise, BR is judged on what is considered to be age-appropriate. In terms of European and American standards, when 2-year-old children have temper tantrums, their behavior is considered to be appropriate, whereas a tantrum by a 30-year-old is considered highly inappropriate.

As participants improvise scenes, they practice behavioral responses to cues given by the other actors that are appropriate to the improvised situation. Scene replays are ways to teach participants that many choices of behavior exist for each situation. Being given permission to act out the wrong way to behave in a situation can be fun as well as instructive. After the scene, participants can discuss why a choice did not work or was an immature choice. Acting out appropriate behaviors allows practice in skills that participants need to develop.

Executive Functions Within Metacognition, Emotional Regulation, and Behavioral Regulation

Initiation

Initiation is the ability to begin a task cognitively and physically through action in the frontal lobes. The frontal lobes send an initiation signal allowing the task to begin. If the frontal lobes are damaged or not fully developed, initiation cannot happen. The non-initiating individual may appear to lack motivation. However, no matter how much an individual wants to initiate a task, without that frontal lobe assistance, initiation cannot happen. The frontal lobes do not become fully developed until at least the age of 24, which is why adolescents often have difficulty initiating projects.

To initiate an action, one must also be able to ignore distractions that get in the way. In addition, successful initiation requires the support of other executive skills like attention, organizing, prioritizing, and inhibition. In fact, few EFs work alone.

The tools we use to help us with initiation—timers, alarms, planners, calendars, and prompts—do not teach initiation. They are tools to alert or remind, but do not create the initiation or motivation for an action. A participant with severe depression is not going to be motivated to get out of bed by an alarm clock; the lack of initiation is not being supported by the frontal lobes. One of the challenges that traditional therapists face is how to motivate initiation in participants with frontal lobe deficits. One of the benefits of the creative arts therapies is that with action methods and support of the group, the frontal lobes can be circumvented by engaging the motor system.

When people have difficulty with initiation, a concrete prompt can engage them. For instance, participants can be asked to choose a postcard or picture that they are drawn to from a collection of diverse images and invent a story or a poem about it. This could be done individually or as a group. Participants could create a scene using three props chosen from a collection of unrelated items as inspiration for the story. The postcard, image, or prop, assigned or chosen, provides initiating ideas for the creation of a character, story, poem, or improvised situation. Tools like alarm clocks can be experienced as punitive, while tools within the creative sphere can be intrinsically motivating.

Inhibition

Inhibition is the ability to stop a cognitive, emotional, or behavioral response. This is not a defense mechanism; it is a conscious, appropriate, thought out response to environmental and social cues within one's culture. A driver cut off by another car who does not erupt in road rage has inhibited emotional impulses. Ruminators often struggle with inhibition. They go over and over and over the same thoughts, trying to work out a problem, but end up thinking in circles. This problem is shared by perfectionists and people with OCD.

There are many drama games which practice stopping or inhibiting actions and initiating others. They are engaging and enjoyable, so participants do not experience shame or judgment while playing them. For "freeze-and-justify," an improvisational scene is started and at any point a member of the group not in the scene can say, "Freeze!" The action stops, and the person who yelled "Freeze!" replaces one of the actors and initiates a new scene. Freezing requires the group members to inhibit their thoughts, behaviors, and emotions in the scene and prepare themselves to initiate a new direction, character, topic, or conflict.

Metacognition, ER, and BR all come together in Marsha Linehan's concept of *wise mind* (1993). This can be enacted (Rubin, 2008, 2015). Wise mind is the metacognitive space where the reasonable or rational mind and the emotional mind become integrated with intuition to become the wise mind. Acting out reasonable mind, emotional mind, and wise mind allows the participant to experience the dysregulation of the emotional mind space and the disconnection of the reasonable mind before integrating them into wise mind. The participant begins to understand not just how to integrate the two minds, but also to experience that the wise mind allows better functioning. The distance that the exercise provides by working in dramatic reality allows the participant to sit in wise mind for longer periods of time without becoming overwhelmed.

Executive Functions Within Metacognition and Emotional Regulation

Self-Reflection

Self-reflection involves being aware of the self and being able to check-in with the self in the present cognitively, emotionally, and behaviorally. It also involves being able to look back at the self over time to evaluate how well or poorly one has functioned. Self-reflection is an ability that many drama therapy participants have not developed. When a parent or teacher asks a young child to think about their behavior, self-reflection begins to develop. If no one is asking these questions, the ability to self-reflect may not develop.

The neurological chemistry of a few diagnoses inhibits the brain functions that allow accurate self-reflection (e.g., schizophrenia, severe anxiety, depression, or the manic phase of bipolar disorder). Individuals who have personality disorders have often developed traits that impede their ability to self-monitor. Nothing chemical or physiological is creating those impairments; their personality traits, such as lack of self-identity, lack of empathy, or fear of looking at the self, lead them to avoid self-monitoring.

Self-reflection also involves being aware of the effect one's behavior has on others. This requires a simultaneous process of seeing the action of oneself in relation to the responses of others and connecting their reaction to the behavior of the self. This ability relates to ER since emotions must be identified in self and others in order to regulate and respond appropriately to them. Someone who cannot self-reflect is not able to inhibit inappropriate behavior.

Drama therapy can be very useful for teaching self-reflection. On the simplest level, discussing any drama therapy intervention afterwards with the group will begin to model self-reflection for participants. There are interventions that build self-reflection. "Emotion mirroring" is one acting exercise that makes participants aware of their own feelings and the feelings of their partner. Analyzing a play and studying character development can enhance this kind of awareness. Having participants journal at the end of a session can also boost self-reflection.

Emotional Attention Set-Shifting

Emotional attention set-shifting allows an individual to use the EF of shifting attention toward or away from a stimulus to regulate emotional response (Johnson, 2009). This skill can be very useful in regulating emotion. An example of shifting away from a negative emotional stimulus: If a girl is afraid of dogs and must walk down a street where a dog is barking from behind a securely fenced-in yard, she can shift her attention from the dog to the flowers growing in the narrow strip of grass between the sidewalk and the street. By doing this she can distract herself and calm down as she walks by the dog.

An example of shifting toward an emotional stimulus: An employee whose creative idea was stolen at work by a colleague could focus on how the creative idea is going to benefit the company to avoid expressing anger or concern at the theft. This can maintain peace and status quo in the office. However, if the employee needs to improve self-assertiveness, it might be more appropriate to shift focus to the theft. To do this, there will be a need to feel the anger, which is an appropriate response to theft of intellectual property, confront the colleague in a calm manner, and seek credit for the idea. In metacognition this ability is called set-shifting, and in ER it is called *cognitive reappraisal* (Hendricks & Buchanan, 2016). Participants who tend to get stuck in emotional responses need to work on this skill.

Emotional attention set-shifting can be practiced by an improvisational game named "calling out emotions" (Emunah, 2020, pp. 205–206). As actors improvise a scene, members of the audience call out different emotions than those being expressed, and the actors must switch how they are playing the scene to the new emotion. For instance, if three robbers are seriously and quietly sneaking up on a bank they want to rob at night, an audience member could call out, "Paranoid," and they might start suspecting each other of setting a trap. Then, if someone else calls out, "Giddy," they might stop suspecting each other and start finding everything that happens hysterically funny.

"Emotional spaces" (Emunah, 2020, p. 176) also provides practice in this skill. Each corner of the room represents a different emotion, perhaps joy, anger, sadness, and fear. When participants are in the sadness area, that emotion is the only one they can express. When they move to a new space, they must shift their emotion.

Executive Functions Within Metacognition and Behavioral Regulation

Task Planning and Organization

Task organization includes planning a task and organizing the materials needed to complete it. Planning prepares for taking on a task. First, the goals for the task must be defined. What is the end result of the task? Then the subtasks are identified and prioritized in their sequence step-by-step.

In order to meet the deadline for the task, the time needed for the completion of each step must be estimated. From those predictions, the deadline for the entire task is set. Working backwards from the deadline, the planner knows when the task must be started. Whether the predictions are correct will depend on previous experience with this type of task, knowledge of the skills involved, and being aware of obstacles that might come up. Organizing the materials for a task is part of the planning. It can happen while the subtasks are figured out or after the planning is completed.

"Embodied life maps" allow participants to plan how to approach a life change in a step-by-step manner by creating a three-dimensional map of how to get from the beginning of the process to the end. Each person thinks through the whole process in detail and verbalizes how to move from one step to the next. Group members watch each other go through the map. If they think the traveler is missing a step or has put a step out of sequence, they can challenge the traveler to think again or offer suggestions. This allows for group feedback to the traveler and provides everyone with additional practice recognizing good planning and organizing.

"Six-word memoirs" require participants to summarize the story of their life or the story of their problem in six words. All the pertinent events have to be boiled down to their essence and organized in a manner that creates a meaningful statement (Fershleiser & Smith, 2008). Later the group member can direct others to act this memoir out, providing practice with sequencing and task monitoring.

Task Monitoring

Task monitoring is an EF used during the process of completing a task. The person must examine the task as it is being completed and the behaviors that are impacting the task. When the task is completed, the final result is evaluated. There are several objectives involved in these three-task monitoring processes.

Examining the Task

Examining the task includes sequencing the actions of the task and keeping track of the time allotted to complete the task. When a task cannot be completed in one sitting, sub-deadlines need to be built into the plan. This requires the person to monitor both time in the present work period and time in the larger context of the project. When group members are involved in a time-limited activity, leaders can provide reports at intervals on the amount of time remaining. These reminders can be followed up after the completion of the task by discussing the need to become aware of the passage of time when working on a project. In terms of projects that stretch over more than one session, therapists can help group members create time planners, organize calendars, or set reminder functions on electronic devices.

Monitoring the Task

Self-monitoring includes all the positive and negative thoughts and behaviors that impact the task, such as negative self-talk, avoidant behaviors, seeking appropriate and timely support, and recognizing strengths and weaknesses related to the task. In the case of timed tests or other time-limited activities, perfectionists run into trouble by spending too much time on details, being critical of their work, or catastrophizing about the outcome of the task. The most effective use of time is first to rough out the whole structure and then go back to fill in the details. Drama therapy interventions can help participants practice letting go of their inner critic through improvisational games or by putting the inner critic in "the empty chair" and telling it to keep quiet for a while. If the issue is avoidance or catastrophizing, the participant could list all the obstacles that might stop work, and an obstacle course could be set up in the room with other group members representing each obstacle. The avoidant participant must get from the beginning to the end of the obstacle course by getting past the obstacles through verbal and physical means.

Evaluating the End Result

Task monitoring also includes evaluating the task for mistakes, and if there are mistakes, making the appropriate corrections. *The Dunning-Kruger effect* is when people have higher opinions of their abilities and/or knowledge than they have in reality (Kruger & Dunning, 1999). This self-evaluating misperception affects the willingness to check a task for mistakes. Those who are nonanalytic tend to overestimate their abilities, while those who are analytic or self-reflective tend to be more realistic or underestimate their abilities (Pennycook, Ross, Koehler, & Fugelsang, 2017).

In order to create a successful intervention, the therapist must distinguish between group members who have an inability to self-evaluate in effortful thought versus those with an unwillingness or disinterest in engaging in self-evaluation. If the participants can be engaged, they will be more willing to be self-reflective and evaluate potential mistakes (Pennycook et al., 2017). Group members who are narcissistic or who are in denial about an addiction may have a conflict in recognizing incorrect answers or actions involved in a task; they are not fully able to monitor tasks without intervention. Interestingly, the more these participants are off the mark in their judgment of themselves and the more invested they are in being right, the more they overestimate themselves (Pennycook et al., 2017). This can be difficult to handle in talk therapy because the therapist is dealing with a resistant participant who is also in denial. By getting participants physically and emotionally engaged and by manipulating the emotional distance the person has to the project, drama therapists can break through denial and entice participants to reevaluate their beliefs about their infallibility. Once this happens, they can begin learning to accurately monitor their thoughts, emotions, and actions.

One example of an intervention that incorporates many aspects of EF, ER, and BR is "the role theatre of life" (Jennings, 1998). The participant creates a metaphorical theatre of their life, identifies all of the roles currently in their role repertoire as well as past roles and roles they are developing, and places the roles in the appropriate space of the theatre. For instance, roles, which are played every day, would be on stage while roles that are not used anymore may be in costume storage. The role theatre of life addresses metacognition, working memory, attention, shifting attention, sequencing, initiation, self-reflection, task planning and organizing, and task monitoring.

Empathy

Empathy is the ability to step outside of one's self to connect with what another is feeling, while still being engaged in one's own life experience. This allows humans to really hear and understand what another person's felt experience is as they tell their story or act it out. This is possible because people often have similar emotional and physical responses. On the physical side, most people have experienced the pain of stubbing a toe or tripping and falling. On the emotional side, most children have been caught lying or disobeying their parents and the shame and guilt of letting their parents down. As humans, we also have the ability to relate to another's experience, even if we have not experienced the same event. In this case we use our imaginations.

As mentioned in Chapter Two, there are two areas in the study of empathy; one group of researchers have explored the concept of cognitive empathy while others have explored emotional empathy (Krznaric, 2014). Some scholars argue that true empathy requires the integration of cognitive and emotional empathy (Staub, 1987). However, there are fMRI studies that have shown that different neural systems are activated for each (Nummenmaa, Hirvonen, Parkkola, & Hietanen, 2008; Lanzoni, 2018).

How empathy is created is not yet clearly understood, but some neuroscientific researchers (Gallagher & Frith, 2003; Gallese, Kesers, & Rizzolatti, 2004; Nummenmaa et al., 2008) theorize that there are mirror neurons in the premotor cortex, limbic system, and the gut that link one person's physio-affective response to the person being observed or interacted with. It is further hypothesized that the mirror neuron system is connected to other parts of the brain, including the frontal lobes and the cerebellum, creating both emotional and cognitive empathy (Gallese, 2016; Gallese et al., 2004; Gallese & Lakoff, 2005; Lanzoni, 2018).

Cognitive Empathy

In simplest terms, cognitive empathy is perspective-taking, a conscious, effortful process that is undertaken to understand another's experience. It often involves comparing one's experience to another's experience to see if it is similar. If the other person seems to be experiencing a physical or emotional event that we have not experienced, we use our imagination to know or hypothesize what the other is going through. At all times in cognitive empathy, one stays with one's own experience, understanding but not experiencing the emotional state of the other.

Cognitive empathy is the easiest type of empathy to teach. "Emotion sculpting" can allow participants to explore what emotions look like physically by observing what others might be expressing visually in their bodies. Of course, not everyone expresses what they are feeling in a visual manner; some people mask their emotions. That aspect of emotional identification needs to be included in the discussion as well. The partner who is being sculpted, embodying the emotion, may have a physiological response to being put into the physical position depicting the emotion. This allows the sculptor and the person being sculpted to learn together from this intervention. *Physiological response* is what happens when actors use Michael Chekov's psychophysical gesture technique (Chekov, 1991; Stanislavski, 1948) or Bloch's (1993) Alba Emoting™ technique. The physical posture, breath pattern, heartbeat, and body tension of an emotion can evoke a physical emotional response.

Affective or Emotional Empathy

For most people, emotional empathy is automatic and unconscious. Emotional empathy is experienced when a person witnesses another having an emotional experience. The witness's body responds emotionally and physiologically to the person being watched. Often the witness micro-mirrors facial expressions or body postures of the person they are observing.

Individuals who empathize too much are said to have empathetic reactivity or empathic overarousal. Professionals who work with trauma, such as therapists, nurses, and doctors, must guard against empathic overarousal by creating clear boundaries, having regular supervision, and taking time for breaks and self-care (Krznaric, 2014). Karla McLaren, a self-identified empath, stresses that highly empathetic people must spend as much time taking care of themselves as they do taking care of others (2013).

Occasionally a drama therapy participant will be empathetically reactive and begin to feel emotionally overwhelmed. The therapist can add more distance to the intervention and work with that participant to create personal boundaries, teaching how to protect themselves. Groups can also be emphatically reactive. This is seen in cases of emotional contagion when everyone takes on the strong emotion of someone in the group. Emotional contagion can be positive or negative. It motivates the desire to respond to others. This is why funders approach their money-raising campaigns through pictures of needy people rather than statistics. In the negative instance of emotional contagion, an angry, charismatic speaker can stir up a riot.

Some participants lack empathy skills rather than feel too much. When dealing with mental illness, alexithymia, personality disorders, and neurocognitive or developmental issues, participants' abilities to recognize their physio-affective response is not highly developed or is muted by the condition. These participants need to improve their emotional empathy skills.

Playback theatre is excellent for developing emotional empathy. This is why playback theatre is often used in school situations where bullying has become a problem or in situations of social injustice where emotional empathy is required. The teller shares a story about a personal experience, then the actors in the troupe improvise the story. The better the playback actors are and the more they can evoke the emotional essence of the story, the more the audience feels empathy with the story and the teller.

Emotional and Cognitive Empathy

Empathy is often intertwined with distance. British dramatherapist John Casson (2004) stated that in order to understand the self/other connection (e.g., empathy), a person needs to be in the middle of the distancing continuum. This allows one to think and feel at the same time, thereby having access to cognitive and emotional empathy. When one is underdistanced, there is loss of the self, and when one is overdistanced, there is isolation from the other's experience; both limit the ability to experience empathy.

In drama therapy, cognitive and emotional empathy are often worked on together. "Doubling" in psychodrama and sociodrama provides practice with both kinds of empathy. In order to double a protagonist, the double must be an empathic witness, or no suggestions will resonate with the protagonist. "Role reversal" also provides practice with both kinds of empathy. When two characters switch roles, they literally switch places, take the other's physical position and perspective, and begin saying the other character's last lines to continue the scene. This provides each actor/character with insight into how the other thinks and feels. After the actors are role-reversed back, they have a better understanding of each other's characters and can communicate and work out problems more empathically. Susan Lanzoni reports in her book *Empathy: A History* (2018) that role-play has been the one method all therapists, peace activists, and social justice advocates have successfully used to teach empathy.

Locus of Control

LOC is a construct that comes from social learning theory, originally proposed by Julius Rotter (1966) and extensively developed over the intervening years by Stephen Nowicki (2016). LOC measures how we perceive what happens to us and whether we believe that we control our lives or if we believe we are controlled by luck, chance, fate, and/or other people.

People who score high in internal LOC believe they can influence what happens to them through their own actions. People high in internal LOC take responsibility for what they have done, can delay gratification, are persistent in solving problems, and tend to be successful in school, work, and life in general. They are willing to continue to practice skills until they have learned them. They are better able to handle a lack of structure because they can create structure for themselves. They also have better outcomes when sick (Nowicki, 2016).

People who score high in external LOC believe they do not have control over their lives and that if they take action to solve a problem, it will not make any difference. People high in external LOC feel helpless, have poorer health outcomes, and poorer achievement at school and work. Research has indicated that poor and oppressed people tend to have high external LOC. They have learned through experience that they are in a one-down position in society and their individual actions will not create much change. In their assessment they are being realistic, not lazy or superstitious. Children and older adults tend to have higher external LOC. Children are more external because they are inexperienced and have not yet learned many skills. Adults tell them what to do and structure their lives for them. Older adults tend to be more external because through aging, losses in life, and declines in health, they have realized they are no longer in control of their lives in the same way they were (or thought they were) when they were younger (Nowicki, 2016).

Measurements at extreme ends of the LOC scale can be problematic. A very high internal score can lead one to be perfectionistic, stressed, anxious, guilt-ridden, and inflexible. To believe you are in complete control is unrealistic and sets up impossible standards that no one can achieve. In our world there are accidents, natural disasters, and other forces like economic recessions and job cutbacks that can be prepared for, but not avoided or controlled. Failure is not a crime; it is one of the ways we learn. If we are afraid to take a risk and fail, we will never grow and ultimately never succeed. By the same token, someone with an extremely high external score can easily become a victim or a pawn, used by others, subservient to them, and easily controlled.

LOC is learned through our life experiences. Children of divorce or from abusive families tend to be more external than children in two parent, conventional families. Children who grow up in poverty tend to be more external than children of middle- or upper-class families. Often birth order makes a difference. Firstborns and only children tend to have more internal LOC while younger children, especially in large families, tend to have more external LOC. There are no big differences based on sex: men and women test similarly (Nowicki, 2016).

Several LOC studies (Felton & Biggs, 1972; Foulds, 1971) utilized gestalt-based therapy techniques with college students. Foulds (1971) led a group of 30 college students using Gestalt techniques in eight weekly four-and-one-half-hour sessions. The students in the group increased their internality while a control group did not. Felton and Biggs (1972) led a group of college students once a week for four weeks in 90-minute sessions. They also showed a change in LOC scores toward internality.

The LOC studies referred to earlier were done back in the heyday of LOC experimentation. However, LOC is not forgotten as an important construct for healthy psychological functioning. In a guest blog post on *Education Week*, Michael J. Hynes (2018), superintendent of schools for the Patchogue-Medford school district in Long Island, NY, writes about how play is related to the ability of children to develop LOC and cites Peter Gray of the Let It Grow Project as saying: "Free play and exploration are, historically, the means by which children learn to solve their own problems, control their own lives, develop their own interests, and become competent in pursuit of their own interests" (as cited in Hynes, 2018, para 5). Hynes then ends with "Let's provide more opportunities in school so children learn how to make decisions and develop an *internal locus of control*" (Hynes, 2018, para 11, emphasis in the original).

Many of the populations that drama therapists work with have external LOC because of their age (children and older adults), diagnosis (depression, schizophrenia, or other mental or physical illness), institutionalization (prison, refugee camp, or orphanage), or other situations of powerlessness (being part of a nondominant group, being sexual trafficked, being homeless, etc.). Many drama therapy interventions are focused on helping participants see the connection between actions and consequences. This can be difficult to teach through discussion, because, unlike math where there is usually only one correct answer, in life there are many choices that can be made. Some choices are better than others; some are terrible. Through playing and replaying scenes in drama therapy sessions, participants can experience those connections and the possible positive and negative outcomes that could result. Instead of actions being seen as hopeless or useless, participants begin seeing them as positive stepping-stones to a better future.

The only way to fail in drama therapy is to refuse to try anything. If a participant makes a negative choice, a learning opportunity is created to explore why it was negative. A scene done in drama therapy is not a real-life situation with real, unchangeable consequences. Participants are in a safe space to fail and figure out what went wrong.

One deficit found in people who are external is poor awareness of nonverbal cues (Nowicki, 2016). They are not clearly aware of how they are expressing their feelings through their faces, gestures, bodies, and tone of voice. They also have a poor ability to read the nonverbal communications of others, causing conflict and misunderstanding between the external person and others. However, many of the drama therapy interventions used in phases one and two can provide practice in understanding nonverbal communications. Participants start seeing the messages others are expressing nonverbally and misunderstand what is being communicated less frequently. They begin to increase interoceptive awareness with their muscles, posture, and other internal sensory processes so they become conscious of their bodies and communicate more clearly to others.

Substance abusers tend to have external LOC and blame their addiction or their drug of choice for their inability to stay sober. While in full-blown addiction, addicts focus on getting their next fix, not on long-term goals. They isolate and distrust others, while also distrusting themselves. They feel at the beck and call of their drug of choice. Once addicts begin working on their recovery, they need to be put in situations in which they can set goals, take responsibility, and prove to themselves that they are capable of change. Studies on alcoholics (Marlatt & Marques, 1976; O'Leary, Donovan, Hague, & Shea, 1975; O'Leary, Donovan, & O'Leary, 1976; Oziel & Obitz, 1975) show that male alcoholics in structured treatment had LOC scores that were more internal than male alcoholics who had never had treatment or had only had detoxification treatment. Drama therapy group can be a place where participants visualize their goals through dramatic sculpts, artwork, or acting out how to achieve what they desire. Then they can practice all the steps and social skills that are necessary in order to get there. This moves from cognitive efforts to embodied work. It is harder to throw away a goal that has been visualized, experienced, and explored how to be achieved.

Conclusion

This chapter discussed some of the components that will go into creating treatment plans. The DSM-5 and ICD-11 pertain to how drama therapists understand diagnosis. As mentioned earlier, many institutions require these coding systems as part of their diagnosis, documentation, and reporting systems. While understanding that diagnosis must be addressed before treatment planning, addressing strengths-based goals is equally, if not more, important. Drama therapists must start where the participants are. Drama therapy effectively builds upon strengths so that a safe therapeutic container for negative emotions and experiences can be built in the early phases of treatment. This allows the group members and the drama therapist to deal more effectively with negative experiences later as treatment deepens, allowing for a corrective experience.

A significant portion of this chapter focused on global functioning as opposed to diagnostic symptoms because drama therapy interventions often work simultaneously on multiple areas. Within the strengths-based philosophy, targeting global outcomes rather than individual symptoms within a diagnosis can be a more effective way to improve the participant's overall life. Global outcomes, such as creativity, spontaneity, SI, EF, empathy, and LOC, all cross multiple diagnostic domains. We will now incorporate information from this and previous chapters in Chapter Four to examine the process of creating a drama therapy treatment plan.

NOTE

1. The ICD-11 was presented to the World Health Assembly for adoption May 2019 and will come into effect on January 1, 2022. This book was written while changes were in process, and online references may no longer be available. Updates will be available in 2022.

SECTION 2

THE DRAMA THERAPY DECISION TREE

4

A Systematic Method of Drama Therapy Treatment Planning

Drama therapists base their therapeutic decisions on the foundational components discussed in Chapters One through Three: group and individual therapy principles and processes, drama therapy principles and processes, diagnostic symptoms, and global functioning. To create clarity on how to systematically utilize all this information, this chapter presents the first part of the drama therapy decision tree: a list of questions for drama therapists to ask themselves when assessing participants and developing initial drama therapy treatment plans. Chapter Five will continue the drama therapy decision tree, focusing on how a drama therapist can make intervention choices. Chapter Six will address evaluating change in the group and, if necessary, revising treatment plans.

These questions represent the most relevant ones that need to be asked when preparing an initial treatment plan. There will be times when certain questions are not applicable to a participant; when not necessary, skip those. Be aware that this list is not exhaustive of everything that might need to be considered: individual circumstances always require additional thought. In addition, certain questions within the decision tree may pertain to an aspect of the treatment plan that is better suited for another mental health professional to address. These kinds of questions should not be skipped over; sometimes when traditional psychotherapy or a medical intervention is employed to address a symptom, there may be a place for drama therapy in preparing for or supplementing the traditional intervention.

An early career drama therapist might ask, "How do I know if I should skip one of these questions?" Think about the diagnosis and the symptoms the participant is experiencing and ask yourself: Is drama therapy appropriate to address any of the treatment goal objectives? For instance, if one participant is having a medication compliance issue, but other people in the drama therapy group are not, the drama therapist might be tempted to ignore that issue in group. However, knowing that the ability to evaluate options and make an informed decision are skills that can be practiced in improvisation, the drama therapist could arrange for the participant to participate in a scene that builds those skills. The scene would not have to be about medical compliance; the same skills can be taught with any kind of decision practice as a character solves a conflict in a scene. Think about the flexibility and breadth of domains, skills, and themes that drama therapy can address; if you can justify a drama therapy intervention as useful, consider answering that question.

All drama therapists work within a team model even when they are in private practice. Within an institution, the drama therapist is one member of the overall clinical team. In private practice, a drama therapist will need to refer participants out to other mental health professionals for certain treatment needs that are beyond their scope of practice (e.g., prescription of medication, career counseling, etc.). This means that a treatment plan sometimes is created by an entire team of professionals working together or by a senior member of the team who may be a psychiatrist, psychologist, or social worker. The team may look to the drama therapist to address certain objectives or goals of the treatment plan. Drama therapists have the ability to navigate between deficit-based and strengths-based models and to address the symptoms of the diagnosis along with the participant's areas of global functioning. These skills make drama therapists valuable to treatment teams.

Answering the questions of the drama therapy decision tree leads to the drama therapist being able to have important conversations with other mental health professionals about how drama therapy can address the treatment goals directly and support the basic skills the participant needs to develop in order to scaffold change. These conversations are necessary to translate between the language of traditional psychotherapy and the language of drama therapy. They help provide understanding about how drama therapy interventions can support traditional interventions. Respect is built when other mental health professionals understand what the drama therapist is bringing to the table and how it relates to what other treatment team members are doing. The best treatment for the participant always comes from a truly integrated, intentional team approach.

Traditional Treatment Planning

The treatment plan guides the therapeutic process. The components of a successful treatment plan are treatment goals and objectives, interventions, and assessment. The first step is identifying treatment goals and objectives and how to achieve them. Then interventions are chosen to implement the objectives. Finally, the outcome of the intervention must be assessed to see if it actually achieved its purpose.

Insurance often uses treatment plans to measure the progress of treatment. Most mental health organizations require carefully documented treatment plans. These, along with written documentation of sessions, support the evaluation of whether treatment goals have been attained.

Getting to a treatment plan is a three-step process: (1) knowing the right questions to ask, (2) identifying what is important in the answers, and (3) given the important information, creating a comprehensive plan. Asking the wrong questions will lead to the wrong goals; hence the need for the drama therapy decision tree. Examining the answers to the right questions leads the clinician to what is relevant and what needs to be prioritized. Also important in treatment planning is realizing what can be worked on at the present time and what cannot be worked on right now. For example, a participant who has borderline personality disorder may have experienced trauma from childhood abuse, but long before that can be dealt with in therapy, the participant needs to learn how to self-soothe and emotionally regulate.

In traditional treatment planning, the therapist identifies the *treatment goals* and *objectives*. Goals are broad, and objectives are specific. In simple terms, if a treatment plan is a map of the treatment, a treatment goal is the description of the destination for therapy, a statement of a desired outcome. A goal is not the process for achieving the outcome. Objectives are specific, measurable, and observable steps to attaining the goal. One way to remember the qualities needed in an objective is to use the acronym STOMO: specific, timely, observable, measurable objectives.

One goal for a participant who has major depressive disorder would most likely be increasing improved mood. One objective for that goal could be that the participant will develop the ability to challenge cognitive distortions. To make the objective more specific, the therapist could say: Participant will identify three cognitive distortions a day and think of one piece of evidence to debate each of those distortions. Once a treatment plan is formulated, the therapist must decide what intervention(s) will achieve those objectives. The intervention used could be from cognitive behavioral therapy, dialectical behavior therapy, or, in our case, drama therapy. Evaluation of the participant after the intervention tells the therapist if the objective has been met.

The wording of treatment plans tends to focus on specific diagnostic symptoms in order to reduce the problems the participant has. This style is used because many traditional therapy approaches come from a deficit-based model. There is a movement toward more strengths-based approaches within humanistic therapies and the development of the positive psychology movement. Even so, the standard paperwork required by insurance companies for treatment plans has not changed from a deficit-based model, so they usually remain framed in deficit-based language.

However, treatment plans do not have to be deficit-focused. With a change of perspective from only addressing individual symptoms to also addressing global functioning issues, treatment approaches can become more holistic.

Drama Therapy Treatment Planning

Being strengths-based, drama therapists take more of a holistic perspective. One of the reasons is that drama therapy interventions naturally address global functioning issues. For example, if a participant with autism spectrum disorder (ASD) has repetitive verbal tics, a traditional treatment plan could identify a goal of reducing repetitive patterns of behavior, and the objectives under that goal would focus on the steps needed to reduce them. The drama therapist would see the verbal tics as stemming from tension, a lack of flexibility and spontaneity, as part of global functioning. The goal chosen could be to increase behavioral choices, and the objectives would focus on the steps needed to increase flexibility and spontaneity. This opens the door to picking interventions that address a variety of symptoms.

Once an objective is identified, the therapist must choose an intervention to address it. Improved emotional regulation (ER) is often a goal in many diagnoses including ASD. A drama therapist targeting ER might have as an objective: Participant will identify four different emotions. The drama therapy intervention could be making human sculptures, first using a partner's body, and then their own, to demonstrate what four different emotions look like. Creating a sculpture with a partner's body helps the participant identify what an emotion looks like as the participant is looking at the sculpt from the outside. Embodying the sculpture helps the participant identify the proprioceptive and interoceptive experiences of the emotion.

Multiple objectives can often be targeted with one intervention instead of using one intervention for each objective. In the beginning of therapy, getting participants to open up and talk can sometimes be difficult and is often an initial treatment goal. Practice in the drama therapy group creating short improvised scenes may help participants feel comfortable being the center of attention, since being a character in a scene takes the focus off themselves and onto the scene partner and the role they are playing. Talking in group then becomes easier.

In targeting a specific goal, say problem-solving, there might be three objectives: Participant will be able to generate alternative options; participant will be able to evaluate alternative options; and participant will be able to implement one of the alternative options. One intervention that meets all three objectives might be to have a small group create a scene involving three props. This task would require the participants to brainstorm solutions, pick a solution for each prop, and actively execute the ideas to act out a story.

Following the intervention, assessment in some form is necessary to determine whether or not the goals and objectives have been met. Agencies and insurance panels often have standardized assessments of goals and objectives that the therapist is required to use. In drama therapy there often is an assessment inherent in the intervention. For example, if a barrier-free theatre production is being used as an intervention for a group to address improvement in social skills, participants must demonstrate a basic level of social skills in order to create, rehearse, and perform a play. If they cannot, rehearsals will fall apart, and "the show won't go on."

Creating Treatment Plans With the Drama Therapy Decision Tree

It is imperative to base goals, objectives, and drama therapy interventions on the diagnosis and presenting problems of the participant. Not only is the diagnosis the focus of what insurance reimburses, it is also what allows for a common language among mental health practitioners. In order to demonstrate how to get from a diagnosis to a treatment plan, we will create a plan for a fictional participant named Jennifer.

The boxes on the following pages present the decision tree questions a drama therapist needs to ask in relation to a diagnosis before creating a treatment plan. The decision tree allows thinking through the diagnosis in a systematic way while taking into account the individual differences of each participant. A therapist must be able to recognize safety concerns (e.g., suicidal ideation or high blood pressure) that need to be prioritized. In addition, a therapist must be aware of skills that need scaffolding. Participants often need to develop primary skills before they can succeed with more complex ones. Safety concerns and scaffolding needs often point the therapist toward where treatment should begin.

Answers to decision tree questions become important data that need to be remembered for when the actual treatment plan is written. Answers may lead to more questions that need to be asked of the participant. Answers can also point out which goals need to be prioritized.

Fictional Participant Description

Jennifer is a 35-year-old, single, African American woman. She grew up in a lower-middle-class household in an urban area with little diversity and was the first member of her family to finish college. There was a strong emphasis put on hard work, morality, and honesty. Her family is Catholic, and she attended Catholic schools on a partial scholarship.

Jennifer was diagnosed with major depressive disorder three years ago and, after participating in cognitive-behavioral therapy (CBT) for eight weeks, felt better. Shortly after this, she began having a glass of wine with dinner to help relax after a stressful day at work. Six months ago, she was passed over for promotion at her job for the third time. She felt angry with her boss and the upper administration; she also felt hopeless about moving ahead in her career. After her initial reaction, she began feeling depressed and worthless. She also experienced insomnia, typically falling asleep between 3 and 4 a.m. She reported that when the alarm went off each morning, she experienced sleep paralysis and was not able to get out of bed. As a result, she was consistently late to work or did not show up at all. When at work, she was so fatigued that she made many mistakes. She also experienced episodes of dizziness and collapsing. About a month ago, she was fired. After being fired, she went to talk to her priest, and he referred her for treatment. Even though she knew how the symptoms for depression felt like, they snuck up on her, as she had been focused on the lost promotion. The psychiatrist gave her a prescription for an SSRI (antidepressant) two weeks ago, but she has not filled it. The psychiatrist referred her to drama therapy.

What Symptoms Is the Participant Experiencing?

- What are the specific criteria of the DSM?
- Which of the specific criteria does the participant meet?
- What are the observable and/or self-reported dysfunctions?
- Are there global treatment symptoms to address (i.e., executive function, locus of control, etc.)?

The Symptoms and Functioning of the Participant

DSM Criteria for Depression

(1) Feeling sad, empty or hopeless most of the day or nearly every day.
(2) Markedly diminished interest or pleasure in all or most all activities most of the day or nearly every day.
(3) Significant weight loss or gain or significant increase or decrease in appetite nearly every day.
(4) Insomnia or hypersomnia nearly every day.

(5) Psychomotor agitation or retardation nearly every day.
(6) Fatigue or loss of energy nearly every day.
(7) Feelings of worthlessness or excessive or inappropriate guilt nearly every day.
(8) Diminished ability to think or concentrate or indecisiveness nearly every day.
(9) Recurrent thoughts of death, recurrent suicidal ideation or suicide attempt. (DSM-5, pp. 160–161)

Specific Criteria Met by Jennifer

Symptoms 1, 2, 3, 4, 5, 6, 7, 8.

Observable or Self-Reported Dysfunctions

Jennifer has had a difficult time participating in group activities. She has made several statements such as, "What's the point?" and "I'm not worth it." She has difficulty making simple decisions. She reports difficulty sleeping and often appears fatigued or sleepy. She has gained 15 pounds in the last three weeks. She does not currently have suicidal ideation.

Global Functioning Treatment Symptoms

Jennifer has an external locus of control (LOC), executive functioning (EF) issues (specifically, metacognition), and low spontaneity.

Questions and Takeaways to Remember about Symptoms and Global Functioning

Enough sleep is a physical and psychological priority for EF, ER, and general safety. Sleep may be a treatment goal that is dealt with by another member of the team, but is something that a drama therapy session can support with relaxation techniques, breathing exercises, and so on. Often participants with depression feel disconnected from others and the world at large; it is important to assess this and see how much of this she is experiencing. Being part of a drama therapy group would help her connect with others like her, so as not to feel like the only person with depression (universality) and could allow her to generate some positive bonds. Participants who ruminate often feel disconnected from their bodies and "all in their heads;" it would be important to check on this with Jennifer. Drama therapy could help get her "back in her body." Jennifer was prescribed antidepressant medication, but is not taking it. If she starts taking it, the treatment team should be aware that sometimes before an antidepressant begins working, suicidal ideation could form. It usually takes four to eight weeks for the medication to start working. The drama therapist should be aware of what Jennifer is reporting during check-ins and discussions and communicate to the treatment team if there are concerns.

What Are Driving the Symptoms?

- Are there physical causes?
- Are there social or economic causes?
- Are the symptoms being reinforced?
- Is the participant on medication for this diagnosis?
- Is the participant on medication for other medical or mental health issues?
- Is there drug/alcohol/caffeine/tobacco use? Contraindications?

Potential Root Causes Driving the Symptoms

Physical Causes

Once a person has had a depressive incident, the brain is more prone to recurrence. Jennifer is up all night, ruminating, and worrying about being fired from her job. Her insomnia is diminishing her ability to think and concentrate. This could lead to accidents while walking or driving. Her lack of sleep could be influencing her weight gain.

Social or Economic Causes

Jennifer experienced institutional racism and sexism prior to the onset of her first and second (current) episodes of depression. She fears she will never have opportunities to improve her life economically, never be promoted beyond middle management, and never be valued for her unique talents, because the system is stacked against her. She struggles with understanding how she can confront the inequality she faces without making her situation worse. Certain aspects of her childhood environment, her mother's parenting style, and her religion (see "Cultural Aspects") hold her back from being able to assert herself. Research has shown a connection between depression and self-silencing in order not to be seen as a "strong black woman" (Abrams, Hill, & Maxwell, 2019). She is currently very concerned about not having an income and worries about becoming homeless. Even though she has family who would take her in if she lost her apartment, up until now she has been an independent career woman. There is a push and pull between staying within a community with a lower socioeconomic status (SES) and rising to a higher one. The possibility of moving back home would bring this issue to the forefront again.

Reinforcement of the Symptoms

Unknown at this time, however, this may need to be explored.

Medication for This Diagnosis

Jennifer has been prescribed medication, but she is not taking it.

Other Medications

No.

Drug/Alcohol/Caffeine/Tobacco Use

Jennifer does not have a drug problem. She has never been a heavy drinker, but as a way to wind down after work, she started to have a glass of wine with dinner. This habit started shortly after the last depressive episode. Alcohol can negatively affect sleep. She does not drink coffee or tea, but does drink caffeinated diet soda all day. This may also affect her sleep. Jennifer does not smoke.

Questions and Takeaways to Remember About Symptom Causes

Could the caffeinated sodas relate in any way to the insomnia? How late in the day is she drinking soda? Could the glass of wine with dinner be throwing off her sleep cycle? Is her physiological response a priority in terms of her physical health? Is she able to apply for unemployment compensation? If so, has she applied? It will be necessary to explore Jennifer's ambivalence about medication for her depression. How much is Jennifer ruminating? There is a need to explore the impact of racism and sexism in her history in terms of her biopsychosocial responses and her desire to address its impact in therapy. Does she feel that her personal experience of racism and sexism is a priority to process in therapy?

Do the Symptoms Allow the Participant to Avoid or Gain Something?

- If the symptoms allow the participant to avoid something, what is it?
- If the symptoms allow the participant to gain something, what is it?
- Can drama therapy address the underlying issue?

Underlying Purposes of the Symptoms

Jennifer has markedly diminished interest in participating in life activities and searching for a new job. She worked very hard at getting a promotion. Her avoidant behaviors now may be allowing her to escape possible rejection in the job search and facing discrimination again in a new place of work. She is experiencing excessive and inappropriate worthlessness. This reaction may be allowing her to avoid feeling angry all the time, which she worries sets her up to being stereotyped as "just another angry black woman."

Can Drama Therapy Address the Symptoms?

Yes, drama therapy could allow Jennifer to play out her anger to express and release it in a safe environment. For example, Jennifer could enact a fictional scene that parallels what she experienced. This could create distance for her, allowing her to have insights into possible actions to take instead in the future. Humor can also be an emotion regulation strategy for depression, because it creates distance from pain and reframes it (Braniecka et al., 2018). There are many drama therapy interventions that can introduce humor into therapy. She could explore future possibilities through scene work and practice dealing with different problems she has previously faced, such as rejection and fear of being assertive, in order to provide a perspective on her problems and help her stand up against discrimination assertively.

Contraindications to Drama Therapy

Drama therapy cannot replace treatment related to medication or her physical health.

Questions and Takeaways to Remember About Drama Therapy

Drama therapy can be a strong motivator for dealing with the anger, diminished interest in life, and avoidant behaviors of depression. When choosing interventions for Jennifer, the drama therapist will want to remember the positive uses of humor and the need for safety in the group, which could be enhanced through distancing techniques. Be aware of the ethnic makeup of the drama therapy group that Jennifer is assigned to so that she does not become the token person of color.

What Cultural Aspects Need to Be Considered With the Diagnosis?

- Cultural aspects and traditions of the participant that need to be considered:
  - Ethnicity/nationality
  - Religious or spiritual affiliation
  - Gender identity
  - Gender expression
  - Sexual orientation
  - Socioeconomic status
  - Educational attainment
  - Work-related identity
  - Political affiliations or beliefs
  - Geographical culture
  - Language
    - Native/secondary language
    - Dialect
    - Localisms
  - Intersectionality of any of the above
- Are there symptoms the dominant culture sees as abnormal, but the participant's culture sees as appropriate behavior?
- Are there behaviors that are being identified as symptoms that really are a representation of being misunderstood or discriminated against by authorities in the dominant culture?
- Are there symptoms outside of the standard diagnostic criteria that are only associated with or normally expressed in the participant's culture related to this diagnosis that also need to be addressed or acknowledged?

Cultural Aspects of the Participant

Cultural Aspects and Traditions to Be Considered in Relation to Symptoms
Jennifer identifies as African American. She has been a target of institutional racism both in terms of work (being passed over for promotions and being fired) and in terms of other previous and current life experiences. There is distrust in the African American community of medical professionals, especially psychiatrists and psychotherapists. Research has shown that the health consequences of systemic racism are passed from one generation to the next: overactive physiological stress response, impacting cortisol levels, insulin levels, the immune system, and serotonin

levels. This leads to higher mortality rates, low birth weights, asthma, obesity, hypertension, heart disease, diabetes, and cancer (Goosby & Heidbrink, 2013).

Jennifer is a member of the Catholic Church and may hold the belief that she should let God handle her problems rather than seeking mental health services. She may feel guilty that she has allowed herself to become depressed again. She did seek help first from her priest and most likely went to the psychiatrist only at his referral. African Americans who identify as Catholic can feel disconnected from their community or be somewhat ostracized since they are not members of AME or Baptist churches, which are often central to the neighborhood. This could increase the feeling of social isolation associated with depression.

Socioeconomically, Jennifer would be considered middle class in relation to the income she received at her old job. She grew up in a lower middle-class family. She was in middle management in her job and desired to move into upper management. Now she sees herself as potentially homeless in a few months if she is unable to find employment. Her family would take her in if she lost her apartment, but she desires to be independent.

Jennifer identifies as a cisgender female. Mass media images across America promote the ideal beauty for women as being extremely thin. Women who do not "measure up" to this image often experience body-shaming. Because of her lack of physical exercise and emotional eating, Jennifer is gaining weight. In addition, patriarchal culture expects women to get married and have children. Jennifer is 35, still single, and childless.

Intersectionality will exist between race, religion and being a single, career-driven, childless, cisgender woman.

Symptoms Participant's Culture Sees as Appropriate

None.

Symptoms Misunderstood by Dominant Culture

It is possible that Jennifer's boss and/or the upper administration of her previous job were intentionally racist or sexist in not promoting her, or it is possible that their bias was unconscious. In either case, their racism and/or sexism was an actual unfair barrier and threat to Jennifer's value as a worker, her livelihood, and her humanity. If at any point she had expressed anger or sarcasm at not being valued on the job and promoted, she most likely would have been stereotyped as "another angry black woman" or as "an angry feminist." This resulted in her "stuffing her feelings" instead of expressing them and avoiding conflict instead of assertively addressing the barriers she sensed were holding her back. Jennifer's symptoms of fatigue and inability to engage in daily activities is often misunderstood as laziness by the dominant culture. Upper management may have misinterpreted her reaction to being denied promotion as an entitlement or a "chip on her shoulder" instead of depression, particularly since she did not communicate the reasons why she was late or slow on the job.

Cultural Symptoms Outside of Standard Diagnostic Criteria

Sleep paralysis when waking up as well as dizziness and collapsing during the day can be symptoms of depression in African Americans (Bell, Dixie-Bell, & Thompson, 1986).

Questions and Takeaways to Be Remembered

Resistance in therapy might be functional as opposed to pathological. It may have developed out of a healthy need to resist racism and sexism or from her Catholic belief that she should be relying on God to provide healing. Jennifer may not have shared her insomnia or emotional struggles with her boss as depression and other mental illness is highly stigmatized by American society in general.

The goal of treatment needs to focus on giving Jennifer back her personal strength and providing her with the skills she needs to overcome the obstacles she encounters. The resistance she may display due to her depression can be dealt with through the drama therapy interventions chosen and may not need to be written into the treatment plan as specific goals to be addressed.

There may need to be a referral made to a career development program to provide her with support in finding new employment. Thought may need to be given to which aspects of career/job hunting are appropriate to deal with in therapy and which are under the auspices of a different provider.

It may be important to assess if there are identity issues that are in conflict. Do the different intersections of Jennifer's cultural background and her life goals interfere with her formation of a clear sense of self? Is there a way to help her find her own voice in therapy?

Initial Treatment Plan for Jennifer

Prioritizing the Symptoms to Be Addressed in an Initial Treatment Plan

After answering the questions just mentioned, an initial treatment plan can be formulated. Not every symptom can be addressed simultaneously. Too many goals and objectives at the same time makes it difficult to focus for the client and the therapist. Additionally, there is a difference between a treatment need and a desire. A treatment need impacts the participant's immediate functioning and safety concerns. A treatment desire may be able to be deferred until the participant has gained some emotional and physical stability. The box that follows outlines questions that can help prioritize what goals need to be addressed in a first treatment plan.

Questions to Identify Initial Goals for Treatment Plan

- Priority: What are the potential harmful consequences that could occur if a particular symptom is not addressed first?
- What symptoms need to be dealt with in order to create an impact on the participant's day-to-day living or to jump-start success/improvement?
- Are there any symptoms that need to be addressed before other symptoms can be addressed (learning skills, scaffolding understanding, or accepting given life situations, etc.)?
- Are there goals that can address multiple symptoms?
- Are there symptoms that need to be addressed now, but must be addressed by a different professional?

First and foremost, the participant must be kept safe, whether that relates to physical or emotional harm that they are facing due to their symptoms. Examples of these types of symptoms could be frightening hallucinations, suicidality, inability to sleep, flashbacks, or manic behavior. These safety goals need to be given the number one priority. In Jennifer's case, sleeping issues are a safety concern. Her insomnia has caused her to be continuously tired and unable to function well during the day, unable to think clearly, or make decisions. Without a change in this symptom, she could potentially harm herself in an accident caused by clumsiness, falling asleep while driving, or losing her balance. Due to these concerns, dealing with insomnia would be an initial treatment goal.

Second, participants often need to experience at least a little positive improvement in their daily functioning in phase one in order to believe that change is possible. When even just a small shift occurs, participants begin to experience hope that life can get better. For Jennifer, being able to sleep through the night will help her overall functioning. In addition, beginning to work on her external LOC will help empower her and encourage her to trust in her own decision making.

Third, certain goals need to be accomplished before others can be taken on. For example, before a participant can regulate emotions, the participant must be able to identify what an emotion is. A goal of exploring whether to take medication will lead to either taking medication for depression or exploring other options, such as exercise, a diet change, or reframing thoughts.

Before Jennifer is able to find her voice and address the racism she has experienced, she will need to regain her belief in her abilities. Steps can be taken toward this goal in phase one. A goal that moves Jennifer toward self-empowerment could address her feelings of helplessness, hopelessness, and worthlessness, her inability to motivate herself to look for a new job, and her need to identify ways to function successfully in situations where she senses racism and sexism are creating barriers in her way.

Goals that might need to be referred to other professionals include Jennifer's difficulties with finding a new job. That may need to be referred out to a career counselor. Depending on the severity of the sleeping issues, she may have to see a medical doctor. A doctor could rule out other medical issues that could involve insomnia, weight gain, and balance problems.

Deficit-Based Treatment Planning Versus Strength-Based Treatment Planning

Typically, treatment plans are created by the primary clinician, which could be a drama therapist, a traditional counselor, or psychologist. The responsibility for creation of the treatment plan depends on the agency. Some agencies will have a full treatment team that includes medical doctors, psychiatrists, psychologists, social workers, creative arts therapists, and so on. In a team-based approach each member is looking at the same treatment plan and deciding who will address each part. Other agencies or practices may have independent clinicians who come together to discuss cases in supervision, but their treatment planning is not based on a team approach. In this situation, the clinician is responsible for addressing everything on the treatment plan, except for items on the plan that may be referred out.

In creating a treatment plan, the therapist has to understand the approach and language of the environment in which the plan is being written. Sometimes the language of the treatment plan is based on the traditional deficit-based model, and sometimes it comes from a strengths-based model. In either case, the plan will be framed in clinical terms. The following team-based treatment plan for Jennifer demonstrates the difference between the two types of approaches.

Rationale for Goal One

Sleep hygiene was identified as a priority goal because of safety concerns. Jennifer needs to learn techniques for falling asleep and staying asleep. Additionally, lack of sleep is impacting Jennifer's overall physical and psychological functioning (irritability, memory, EF, focus, etc.).

Goal One (Deficit-Based): Insomnia symptoms will be reduced.
Goal One (Strengths-Based): Participant will develop a sleep hygiene plan.

> **Objective One (Deficit-Based):** Participant will identify aspects of her sleeping environment that interfere with sleep.
> **Objective One (Strengths-Based):** Participant will identify three environmental sleep hygiene factors that would encourage sleep.

Objective Two (Deficit-Based): Insomnia-inducing environmental factors will be removed or changed.
Objective Two (Strengths-Based): Participant will implement the three environmental sleep hygiene factors.

Objective Three (Deficit-Based): Participant will identify life and psychological activities, which block sleep and stop doing them before bed.
Objective Three (Strengths-Based): Participant will demonstrate three relaxation and breathing techniques for sleep.

Rationale for Goal Two

The purpose of goal two is to address Jennifer's symptoms of depression. People who are depressed often feel disconnected from their own bodies, from other people, and from the world in general. When participants get "out of their head" and "back into their body," rumination often decreases, as do other symptoms of helplessness and hopelessness. Group treatment, in particular, can help participants connect with others and feel less isolated.

Goal Two (Deficit-Based): Participant will decrease depressive symptoms.
Goal Two (Strengths-Based): Participant will develop better mind-body connection.

Objective One (Deficit-Based): Participant will reduce time spent being inactive.
Objective One (Strengths-Based): Participant will physically engage by participating in drama therapy group warm-ups each session.

Objective Two (Deficit-Based): Participant will reduce time spent in isolation.
Objective Two (Strengths-Based): Participant will participate in drama therapy group by joining in discussions at least twice each session.

Objective Three (Deficit-Based): Participant will complete a symptom tracking sheet once a day.
Objective Three (Strengths-Based): Participant will complete a positive behavior-tracking sheet once a day.

Rationale for Goal Three

The purpose of goal three is to address locus of control (LOC). This will help Jennifer begin to separate the institutional racism she has faced from her worth as a human being and understand what can be controlled and what cannot be controlled. (In "treatment-ese" this might be written as "participant will examine workplace disparities related to her race.")

Goal Three (Deficit-Based): Participant will reduce self-blaming.
Goal Three (Strengths-Based): Participant will increase internal locus of control.

Objective One (Deficit-Based): Participant will identify self-blaming or self-negating statements.
Objective One (Strengths-Based): Participant will identify accurate self-affirming statements.

Objective Two (Deficit-Based): Participant will reduce self-blaming and self-negating statements by 20%.
Objective Two (Strengths-Based): Participant will increase accurate self-affirming statements by 20%.

Objective Three (Deficit-Based): Participant will reduce statements of helplessness by 30%.
Objective Three (Strengths-Based): Participant will verbalize when she experiences her contributions to the group have been accepted or minimized by others.

Rationale for Goal Four

The purpose of goal four is to address decisions around medication compliance. Jennifer needs to discover what is getting in the way of taking her medication. If appropriate, she needs to create motivation for taking medication.

Goal Four (Deficit-Based): Participant will take medication.
Goal Four (Strengths-Based): Participant will make an informed decision regarding taking medication for depression.

Objective One (Deficit-Based): Participant will identify obstacles that impede taking medication for depression.
Objective One (Strengths-Based): Participant will identify reasons for and against taking medication for depression.

Objective Two (Deficit-Based): Participant will create a plan to address identified obstacles to medical compliance.

Objective Two (Strengths-Based): Participant will make an informed decision about whether to take medication for depression.

> ### Is Drama Therapy Appropriate to Address the Treatment Goals?
>
> - What is the rationale for why/how drama therapy would be useful for these goals and objectives?
> - Is there research that supports using drama therapy for this diagnosis?
> - Does the drama therapist have experience using drama therapy with this diagnosis? If not, where is there information? Who could supervise/consult?
> - If this is group therapy, do participants in the group have more than one diagnosis?
>   - If this will cause a problem, how can that best be dealt with?

Is Drama Therapy Appropriate to Address Symptoms?
Yes.

Rationale

The physical activity, social interaction, humor, and fun of the drama therapy group will energize and motivate Jennifer and connect her to other people. Laughter and play will also change her neurochemistry and help lift her mood. The other members of the group are also depressed or anxious, so she will realize she is not alone in feeling this way. Warm-ups and closures often include teaching relaxation and breathing skills, and these would definitely be included in a group with depressed and anxious participants. Role-playing situations that she is facing in her life may provide new ideas for how to overcome frustrating situations, deal with job interviews, address racism, motivate herself to get up in the morning, find new activities and interests to become excited about, and so on.

Research That Supports Using Drama Therapy for Depression

Bornmann, Mitelman, & Beer, 2007; Chapman, 2014; Hamamci, 2006; Keisari, & Palgi, 2017; Mehdi, Sen Mazumdar, & Sen, 1997; Mehdi, Sen, & Sen Mazumdar, 1997; Moore et al., 2017; Terzioglu & Ozkano, 2018.

Does the Drama Therapist Have Experience With the Diagnosis?

If the answer is no, and a referral to another drama therapist with experience is not possible, supervision or consultation is crucial. It is not enough to read up on the diagnosis and methods of using drama therapy with the diagnosis, although this is helpful and important to do. The drama therapy community is very open and willing to share. A request for consultation or supervision made through the dramatherapy listserv or other social media platforms will most likely result in a drama therapist reaching out. Dual supervision with a drama therapy supervisor about the intervention(s) being used and a traditional psychotherapist who has experience with the population can also be helpful.

Considerations: Are There Multiple Diagnoses in the Drama Therapy Group?

Participants in the group will have diagnoses of anxiety and/or depression. There is no anticipation that this will cause problems.

Ongoing Treatment Planning

This chapter is focused on the first treatment plan created as a participant enters therapy. As the participant progresses, changes will be made in treatment plans due to the phase of treatment the participant is in and due to goals/objectives having been met. When changing or revising a treatment plan, the same process of questions and evaluation of the participant and current symptoms and needs must be done. Each phase has basic goals that must be accomplished so therapy can move forward (see Chapter One). These phase goals must be built into the work and not forgotten. For instance, in phase one a therapeutic relationship must be created between participant(s) and therapist. The participant must also invest in treatment, or no work will be accomplished. These basic goals may seem obvious, but overenthusiastic therapists can forgo important building blocks that allow trust and safety to be developed to fast-forward into deep work that the participant is not prepared for. When this happens, participants often stop coming to therapy or begin to resist treatment.

Treatment plans change over time because participants achieve goals and objectives listed in them. This does not necessarily mean that the whole treatment plan must be redone. It may be that new objectives need to be added to further or deepen a goal. It may be that an objective did not align with a goal, and the therapist is not aware until actually working with the participant. In that case, the objective needs to be revised or replaced. As participants move into later phases, additional goals can be added that the participant and therapist recognize as important to address, but which could not be addressed until other work was done.

Conclusion

No matter the orientation of the treatment plan (deficit- or strengths-based), drama therapists must be able to connect the goals and objectives of the plan to the appropriate drama therapy interventions that will actively create the desired outcome. Chapter Five continues the drama therapy decision tree to demonstrate the bridge between treatment planning and treatment intervention. The tools available to the drama therapist in terms of intervention include all of the creative methods of drama therapy: words, dialogue, action, spatial relationships, movement, roles, role reversals, performance, and more. In essence, creativity is the bridge used to cross the divide between diagnosis and treatment.

5

A Systematic Method for Choosing Drama Therapy Interventions

Chapter Four focused on diagnosis questions of the drama therapy decision tree and how to create a treatment plan. Therapy cannot begin until the goals and objectives for treatment are developed. Drama therapy was identified as an appropriate intervention for many of the objectives in the treatment plan of our fictional participant Jennifer. A drama therapist can use the next part of the drama therapy decision tree to determine which interventions to use. Jennifer, the fictional participant in Chapter Four, and her treatment plan will continue to be used for illustrating how questions might be answered.

Phase

The phase of treatment a participant is in will be important in determining what interventions would be appropriate or inappropriate. First-time drama therapy participants in phase one may not feel safe to play actively with strangers in a group. They often experience what is called *the spotlight effect* (Gilovich, Medvec, & Savitsky, 2000) or *imaginary audience* (Elkind, 1967) and become so worried about what others are thinking about them that they become inhibited. In actuality, everyone in the group is inwardly focused, worrying about what others are thinking about them. Part of the process of phase one is getting past the spotlight effect in order to become comfortable with being seen by others and being integrated into the group. Skills are built as the participant moves through treatment. Obviously, participants will be more willing to engage fully after they have already developed appropriate skills, such as the ability to invent dialogue, listen to scene partners, and derole themselves from the character they played in scenes.

Jennifer is again our sample participant in this chapter. See Chapter One to review the typical emotional and behavioral signs displayed by participants in each phase of treatment. See Chapter Four to review Jennifer's symptoms and treatment plan.

What Phase of Treatment Is the Participant in?

- Has the participant been in drama therapy before?
- What emotional and behavioral signs does the participant exhibit?
  - Which phase do these emotional and behavioral signs fit into?
  - Are there treatment goals that need to be addressed for the participant specific to the phase?
- If doing group treatment, is the group starting now, or is it an ongoing/open group?
  - If the participant is joining an open group, are participants in multiple phases? If so, how do you plan to deal with that?
- What issues addressed in this phase are part of normal group development that do not need to be specifically addressed in the participant's treatment goals (i.e., developing a therapeutic relationship, developing trust between group members, understanding group rules, etc.)? These issues will need to be taken into consideration when choosing an intervention.

Important questions to keep in mind during the course of a phase:

- What are typical signs that the participant/group is ready/not ready to move to the next phase?
- What are signs that the participant/group has regressed to a previous phase?
  - Does the therapist know why this has happened?
  - Does this regression impact treatment goals or intervention choices?

Using this information, identify the phase of treatment the participant/group is in.

What Phase of Treatment Is the Participant in?

Has Jennifer Been in Drama Therapy Before?

No.

What Emotional and Behavioral Signs Does Jennifer Exhibit?

She demonstrates a lack of trust by only sharing minimally, she is not connecting with other people (isolating), and she expresses hopelessness.

Phase in Which These Emotional and Behavioral Signs Fit
Phase one.

Treatment Goals for Jennifer Specific to the Phase
Developing trust, instilling hope, connecting with other group members.

Is the Group Starting or Is It an Ongoing (Open) Group?
Just starting.

If Joining an Ongoing (Open) Group, Are Participants in Multiple Phases?
N/A.

Phase Issues and Behaviors

Phase Issues That Are Part of Normal Group Development
Development of therapeutic relationship, development and internalization of group norms and rules.

Behaviors Indicating the Group Is Ready to Move to the Next Phase
Group members have internalized rules and norms and are following them, have begun to develop trust with each other and the therapist, report feeling safe, interactions demonstrate openness, respect, and caring for others.

Signs Jennifer/Group Has Regressed to a Previous Phase
Missing group therapy sessions, refusing to participate, monopolizing the conversation, acting out hidden agendas.

If the Group Has Regressed, Does the Therapist Know Why This Has Happened?
N/A because the group is just starting.

Does This Regression Impact Treatment Goals or Intervention Choices?
This question is not applicable because the group is just starting.

Phase of Treatment Decision

Jennifer is in phase one.

Outside Influences Impacting the Treatment Process
• Are there any outside influences impacting the participant in personal/work life? • Are there any potential group dynamic issues: o Open versus closed group o Attractions between participants o Animosities between participants

Influences Impacting Treatment Process

Outside Influences
Jennifer is having difficulty with work-life balance, unemployment, money worries due to unemployment, family responsibilities (Jennifer's mother is ill), transportation issues (Jennifer's car is old), and the weather (cloudy, rainy, and cold) impact her willingness to get out of bed.

Potential Group Dynamic Issues
The group will be a closed group. The group has many strong personalities in it. Jennifer is easily irritated by people who swear, take the Lord's name in vain, or make racist or sexist comments.

The Interaction of Diagnosis and Phase

Diagnosis and phase both impact how participants function in treatment. Individuals who are depressed will most likely feel isolated and lonely. The initial stage of treatment may last longer, because it may take longer to develop trust and get past the apathy created by depression. When designing interventions for this diagnosis, therapists need to take into consideration that the group may be in phase one longer and may need more trust-building exercises that do not involve taking initiative or require participants to reach out to others in the group. An example of such an exercise would be a simple name game that only requires people to say their first name to the person on either side of them, as opposed to learning others' names, and pass them back and forth.

In some instances, certain types of interventions would be contraindicated because of diagnosis, and certain interventions that are typically considered phase one or phase two might need to wait for later phases. For instance, participants who have been sexually abused might not feel comfortable with games involving touch. "Trust falls" might fall into the same category. A "blindfold walk" might require more trust than participants are ready for. "Blindfold walks" or "trust falls" might be more appropriate for a phase five ritual for participants who have been sexually abused. For groups with different diagnoses, like Jennifer's, touch in games in phase one could help connect group members.

The Interaction of Diagnosis and Phase of Treatment

- How does the current diagnosis present in this phase of treatment?
  - What interventions might be useful for this diagnosis in this phase?
- How does the current diagnosis present differently in different phases of treatment?
  - What interventions, that might typically be done in the current phase, need to be saved for a later phase, or not done at all?
  - What interventions would be contraindicated in certain phases?
- Are there issues in the diagnosis that could cause difficulty in a specific phase (i.e., dependent personality disorder causing difficulty in termination phase?)
- What issues involved in the diagnosis might impact the length of the phases?

Interaction of Diagnosis and Phase of Treatment for Jennifer

How the Current Diagnosis Presents in This Phase of Treatment

Depressed participants typically have flat affect, low energy, feel helpless, and hopeless. (If this sounds like the diagnosis, it is because no treatment has happened yet in phase one.)

How the Current Diagnosis Typically Presents in Different Phases of Treatment

As participants begin to improve, their affect becomes more animated, their sleep patterns improve, and their energy becomes stronger. They become more connected to their bodies. They begin to gain more perspective on their problems. The goal in treatment then becomes to help develop solutions to those problems.

Issues in the Diagnosis That Could Cause Difficulty in a Specific Phase

In phase one, developing initiative and spontaneity are very difficult for participants who are depressed. In phase five, participants could worry about their depression coming back and might need to practice identifying signs of a new cycle starting and practices they could do on their own to deal with it.

Contraindications With Interventions in Phase One

Using psychodrama or a drama therapy intervention could require sharing deep personal information before trust and communication has been developed.

Issues in Diagnosis Impacting the Length of Phase One

Because Jennifer and the rest of the group have depression and anxiety, they might need more time in phase one to connect with each other and develop trust. They may also need more time in phase two to gain confidence in their acting abilities.

Psychological Distance of Individual/Group

As discussed in Chapter Two, distance is an important concept in drama therapy. Distance can be envisioned as a continuum from underdistanced (over connected to emotion/disconnected from thinking) to overdistanced (disconnected from emotion/over connected to thinking). In the middle of these two positions is a state of balance where the person can think and feel equally. Drama therapists often term this *aesthetic distance*. There are many places on that continuum that people can be from moment to moment.

While participants typically have a specific set of symptoms with a given diagnosis, each one is a unique individual and will have a unique background and personality. One of those individual aspects is how generally emotionally responsive the participant is to events and people. A generally underdistanced person will tend to be more emotionally reactive or responsive to people, places, and things. People with a more overdistanced style would be inclined to speak of experiences and reactions more abstractly and metaphorically. They would talk in generalities and give nonpersonal examples. They may need concrete props, costumes, and activities to pull them toward emotional expression. These concrete objects and interventions help keep them anchored mindfully in the present and in their body.

Despite a predisposition to an emotional style, on any given day, participants will be in a specific emotional place depending on what has happened that day. A typically underdistanced participant might have been in a minor car accident on the way to the group and may enter the room in a very emotional state. On the other hand, the same participant, trying out a new medication, could have a flattened affect and behave more distantly than normal. In each case, the drama therapist will want to use the warm-up to achieve a balance in their psychological distance.

Participant's Overarching Predisposition for Psychological Distance

- Is the participant typically intellectual and unemotional most of the time?
- Is the participant typically highly reactive and emotional most of the time?
- Is the participant relatively balanced between emotion and thought most of the time?

Overarching Predisposition of the Participant

When not depressed, Jennifer is usually a balanced individual. Normally she feels deeply and expresses her emotions verbally and physically in a grounded and appropriate manner; however, her depression symptoms (dizziness, lack of sleep, lack of focus, helplessness and hopelessness, etc.) have made her behavior more overdistanced. As a result, she is being less expressive than normal.

Emotional Regulation Abilities of the Participant and Group

- If the participant/group is typically under- or overdistanced, does this need to be added as a treatment goal?
    - o If yes, what is the urgency? Does a treatment goal need to be added immediately to the treatment plan, or can it wait until other goals have been addressed?
- What is the participant's/group's psychological distance upon arrival at the group today?
- Is something different about the participant's/group's emotional regulation today?
    - o If so, what is different?
    - o What is the reason?
        - ▪ Do they know?
        - ▪ Do you know?
- Are you able to adjust the participant's/group's distance through the warm-up?
    - o If not, how can you address this distancing challenge?

Emotional Regulation

Emotional Regulation Abilities of the Participant
Jennifer has the skills to regulate her emotions, but in trying to function within her workplace where she experienced racism, she started trying to block or ignore her emotions. Now because she is depressed and experiencing insomnia, her emotional regulation abilities are compromised further.

Does This Need to Be Added as a Treatment Goal?
Yes.

How Soon Should It Be Added?
Not immediately. Phase one interventions may naturally help adjust her regulation abilities. Wait and in phase two come back to readdress this question.

Is Something Different With the Participant's Emotional Regulation Today?
Yes, Jennifer's car is in the shop, and she got caught in a downpour at the bus stop on her way to the group.

What Is Different?
She seems to be agitated and distracted.

Is She Aware of the Reason?
Yes.

Emotional Regulation Abilities of the Rest of the Group in General
They tend to have a difficult time regulating their emotions.

Is There Something Different With the Group's Emotional Regulation Today?
Yes, there has been flooding in the city because of heavy rain, and the group has had to take detours to get here. Some got wet on their way to and from their cars.

What Is Different?
They seem to have more difficulty regulating their frustration tolerance.

Are They Aware of the Reason?
Yes, they are aware, as are the facilitators who had to deal with the flooding as well.

Can Therapist Adjust Distance Through Warm-up?
Yes, the therapist will spend more time in warm-up, if needed, until the participants are calm and able to focus.

The Interaction of Diagnosis, Phase, and Psychological Distance

Diagnosis, phase, and psychological distance interact with each other. Together they can influence what aspects of the diagnosis should be focused on in certain phases, the length a treatment phase needs to be, and the participants' engagement or regression in treatment. A mistake that early career clinicians often make is focusing on one of these areas and forgetting that they interact with each other. All the knowledge in the world about the diagnosis, phase of treatment, or psychological distancing as separate entities will not lead to choosing the appropriate intervention if the interaction among them is ignored.

In phase one, participants need to develop trust and safety first. Diagnoses, such as anxiety disorder, social phobia, eating disorders, or post-traumatic stress disorder (PTSD), will require more time developing trust in early phases, while participants whose safety needs are met more easily may move through early phases faster. By the same token, there are participants who because of skill deficits related to their diagnosis, such as individuals with autism spectrum disorders (ASD) or intellectual or developmental disability (IDD), need more time in early phases to develop better functioning in communication and emotional regulation before moving to more complex, insight-oriented work. Equally, older adults with normal cognitive functioning often want the connection, socialization, and creativity that early phases can offer and may not need deeper explorations.

Conversely, there are participants, such as recovering substance abusers, people with borderline personality disorder, and people struggling with grief and loss, whose diagnostic symptoms need to be addressed at a deeper level (phases three and four) in order to consider therapy effective. This does not mean that therapists should jump to those phases before the participants are prepared to work together appropriately. To work through those deep issues, participants will need to have clear boundaries, ego strength, and the ability to respect each other.

Be aware that participants with diagnoses like dependent personality disorder or substance abuse may try to extend treatment once they are in phase five. They worry about the loss of the support of the group and the therapist. They can sabotage termination by bringing up new symptoms in order to take the group back into phase four so that treatment can continue.

Psychological distance and phase impact which symptoms of the diagnosis can be focused on. With a participant who has PTSD, the therapist would need to focus first on developing trust, a therapeutic relationship, and a sense of safety and security before addressing symptoms like flashbacks. If a participant with PTSD in phase one or two has a flashback, it could be accidental or caused by the intervention. The trigger could be environmental, if there were a sudden, loud noise or a smell associated with the trauma. If it is being caused by the intervention, then the therapist has not paid attention to the diagnosis, phase, and psychological distance needs of the participant. Planning a warm-up that involves loud noises, such as “bang!” or “zip-zap-zop,” could be contraindicated, as the chances of creating a flashback are significant.

A significant shift in psychological distance in participants and group can be caused by the interaction of diagnosis, phase, and psychological distance. This is true whether the group has moved in the direction of underdistance or overdistance. For instance, regression in psychological distance and behavior could be caused by a group’s fear of the unknown as they start to transition to a new phase of treatment. Individuals can regress when experiencing appropriate therapeutic changes in phases four and five, because they fear who they might become if they change their behavior. They worry that if their identity changes, they will not know how to function in the world. Many recovering addicts drop out of treatment or get high when faced with moving out of a treatment facility, because they have no faith that they will know how to live clean and sober. When a group regresses, it can be helpful to go back to the type of work that was done in earlier phases to allow the group to feel safe again and regain emotional/behavioral control. The drama therapist could also address the regression directly through an intervention, such as goal setting through “sculpting goals”, “past/present/future sculpting” or a “future projection” in a sociodrama.

The Interaction of Diagnosis, Phase of Treatment, and Psychological Distance

- Is the participant/group under- or overdistanced because of:
  - Medication
  - Diagnosis
  - Typical psychological distance

- Is the psychological distance related to the current phase?
  - Just beginning
  - Transitioning between phases
  - Nearing termination
  - Terminating

Interaction of Diagnosis, Phase of Treatment, and Psychological Distance

Reasons for Over/Underdistance
Jennifer and the group as a whole are overdistanced from the depression and the medications they are taking which "dulls" them out. They could also be underdistanced because of their diagnosis.

Issues Related to Phase
The group is in phase one. They could be overdistanced because they do not know/ trust each other yet and are unsure of this "drama thing."

The Drama Therapy Pie

As discussed in Chapter Three, the drama therapy pie arranges interventions along two different axes: from fictional to nonfictional and from presentational to process-oriented (i.e., rehearsed and shared with an audience versus done through improvisation within the group). Using the pie allows the drama therapist to integrate the diagnosis, phase, and psychological distance needs of the participants to determine the aesthetic distance requirements for the intervention chosen. The following are questions that can help determine which general direction would be the most appropriate and effective way to go.

Choosing an Appropriate Intervention

Fiction or Nonfiction Interventions

- Is the participant/group better able to work with fiction (acting through metaphor/distance) than nonfiction (acting out their own lives)?
- Does the participant/group have enough reality testing to remain psychologically intact if working on traumatic or highly emotional material about their lives?
- Is there enough trust and respect in the group to work with nonfiction material in terms of the vulnerability that comes with personal disclosure?
- What kind of setting are you in?
    - o If in a prison, jail, or detention center, what are the contraindications of nonfiction work?
        - ▪ Disclosure by the participant of crime that must be reported?

    - Participant disclosing information to an "enemy" inside or outside the group (inmate or staff) that could be used against them?
    - Other?
  - In an educational setting, a drama therapist's contract is often focused on psychoeducational goals rather than therapeutic ones, and often class periods are between 45 and 60 minutes. Fictional work tends to provide more containment so students can transition quickly from group to academic class. What is your situation?
  - In long-term residential settings (i.e., treatment centers, nursing homes, etc.), trust may have already been established among residents, and ongoing staff could provide safe containment to help process issues between therapeutic groups. Nonfictional work benefits from the continuity provided by long-term groups. What is your situation like?

Fictional or Nonfictional Interventions

Jennifer's group would be served better in phase one with fictional interventions. The group is very inhibited and depressed, so fictional interventions will help them address issues that feel painful through distance via metaphor. Fictional interventions often involve humor, which is another way of providing distance. Jennifer is dealing with issues of institutional racism. Through the distance fictional drama therapy provides, she can begin to see a wider view of the obstacles facing her and perhaps discover solutions for herself that she could not see while in the midst of the discrimination.

Process-Oriented or Presentational Interventions

- Is the group open or closed? If the group is open, it will be very difficult to create, rehearse, and perform a play since members of the group will change.
- Would the participant/group be able to handle presenting a play in front of an audience?
- Do participants have the social skills to work with each other in rehearsals?
  - If social skills need to be worked on, would rehearsals provide enough practice in working with others?
- Do participants have the emotional regulation to deal with nerves and stage fright?
  - Is sharing the participant's/group's story part of the healing that needs to happen?

- o Have the participants processed the emotional material to be included in the play enough so that they would not be overwhelmed by a new discovery about themselves during the performance?
- o Are there diagnoses in the group where having a wider audience (if doing a play) would be contraindicated, for instance, for participants who are histrionic or attention-seeking?
- o Do the participants have enough ego-strength to deal with the rehearsal and performance process?
- o If autobiographical, does the material being presented in a play have aesthetically pleasing aspects that would be accessible to an audience?
    - Autobiographical or solo performance requires more ego-strength than a fictional or group performance.
    - All plays inherently have a level of fiction and distance, depending on the use of metaphor to express emotional truths. The use of metaphor supports participants who have less ego-strength.
- o Is there a space in which you can perform?

- Are there ethical concerns in having participants perform?
    - o Are there Health Insurance Portability and Accountability Act (HIPAA) concerns or permissions needed regarding participants performing for each other or a larger audience?
    - o Are there issues of confidentiality, such as parental or guardian permission in order to perform?
    - o Are participants the survivors of domestic abuse who need their location kept secret from their abusers?
- Does the aesthetic distance inherent in the type of performance intervention fit with the group needs?
- Would the participant/group do better with process-oriented work?
    - o Do you have enough time to spend in self-discovery and play development (if it is a devised play), or would you need to jump right into mounting a production?
    - o Do you have participants who would not want to perform in a play?
        - ▪ Too young
        - ▪ Not confident enough
        - ▪ Not enough emotional regulation
- Are the issues that need to be worked through severe? If so, staying focused on process might be more useful.
- Life-drama connection (i.e., talking about the intervention afterwards):
    - o Can the participant/group readily understand the life-drama connection, or does it need to be made concrete for them?
    - o Do you want to focus the discussion on the process of the drama therapy work, the outcome of the drama therapy work, or both?

Process-Oriented or Presentational Interventions

Jennifer's group would do better with process-oriented work at the beginning. There are participants who currently would be too shy and lacking in confidence to want to perform. They might drop out of the group if they thought they would have to be in a play. In addition, the mental health organization at which the group is being held does not have a performance venue. However, if participants later indicate a desire to perform, perhaps a short sharing could be created.

What Kind of Embodiment Do the Participants Need?

- Self:
  - Does the participant need hands-on practice/rehearsal to incorporate skills?
  - Does the participant need to be embodied in order to understand or gain insight?
  - Does the participant need to learn give-and-take with other group members?
- Others:
  - Will watching others' enactments provide enough distance for the participant to understand what is going on?
  - Will watching others' enactments provide opportunities for the participant to learn through the observation process?
- Objects (Props, Costumes, Masks, Drawings, etc.):
  - Are objects needed in order to engage participants in therapy?
  - Are objects needed to ensure metaphor (distance) for participants?
  - Are objects needed to ensure understanding (concreteness) for participants?
  - Are objects needed to ensure focus/attention of participants?

What Kind of Embodiment Does Jennifer Need?

Embodiment would be important because with depression and anxiety, participants become physically inactive. Getting back into her body and out of her head would help Jennifer feel more in control and able to make her own decisions. The frontal lobes become reengaged as the process of embodied cognition connects the motor cortex (and accompanying mirror neurons), cerebellum (involved in balance and movement), and the prefrontal cortex (Gallese, 2016; Gallese & Cuccio, 2018; Gallese, Kesers, & Rizzolatti, 2004). Watching others enact situations in which they are overcoming obstacles will help Jennifer see that she is not alone and may help her make connections between their struggles and her own. Objects will provide a sensory experience, which may help embody her and provide opportunities to create concrete metaphors in scenes.

The Interaction of Diagnosis, Phase, Psychological Distance, and the Drama Therapy Pie

Diagnosis, phase, and psychological distance interact with each other and the drama therapy pie. The difference between the previous interactions discussed have to do with the interaction between psychological distance (of the participant) and aesthetic distance (involved with the intervention). The diagnosis, phase, and drama therapy pie impact the choice of intervention while simultaneously providing for the in-the-moment psychological aspects of the participant. The therapist is assessing the participant and group in terms of the trees (where they are in the moment) and in terms of the forest (the bigger picture: where they are headed).

The Interaction of Diagnosis, Phase, Psychological Distance, and Drama Therapy Pie

- Interventions:
  - What interventions are effective in the current phase of treatment?
  - Given those interventions, which are appropriate considering the diagnosis of the participant?
  - Are there specific distance needs?
- Do you want the intervention's aesthetic distance to match or balance the participant's current psychological distance?
  - What type of embodiment does the participant need?
  - Should interventions be fictional or nonfictional?
  - Can this be addressed through the warm-up or will more of the session need to be adjusted to create balance?
  - How much of the life-drama connection needs to be addressed in discussions about the intervention during closure?
- What additional issues relating to diagnosis can be addressed in different phases as treatment progresses for the participant?
  - Can nonfictional interventions be used?

- o Does metaphor provide a wider/more complete view through which participants can see and address their dilemmas?
- Can the level of discussion about interventions become more abstract, less distanced, or more personal as participants develop insight, or due to diagnosis does discussion need to remain concrete and distanced?

Useful Interventions

In phase one spontaneity may be low, so warming up the group at the beginning is essential. "Yes, and ...," "fortunately/unfortunately," "mirroring," "the winds are blowing," and "freeze-and-justify" would be several of the many appropriate interventions to use to develop trust and group cohesion as well as to reintroduce play. In terms of the group of depressed participants that Jennifer will be part of, interventions involving touch to help break isolation and create connection could be helpful in both phases one and two. Most of the interventions would need to be energizing and connecting experiences without deep role development.

Possible Contraindicated Interventions

"Mirroring" might be threatening to someone who is depressed. Mirroring each other might make both partners feel more depressed. The therapist would need to consider how to run this intervention, perhaps using a variation like "emotion mirroring" where participants are asked to act out a variety of emotions. Improvisations like "freeze-and-justify" may require too much energy, initiation, and shifting of attention for participants to jump in quickly.

Aesthetic Distance Needed From Intervention

Typically, depressed people are either underdistanced or overdistanced, so the aesthetic distance of the interventions chosen most likely will need to balance their psychological distance at the beginning of the session. The majority of this group is overdistanced, as is Jennifer; however, there will be days when people arrive in an underdistanced state. The warm-up can address this as drama games tend to create aesthetic distance and pull people to the middle of the continuum. If all else fails, singing can balance a group. The process of singing as a group releases oxytocin and dopamine, both neurochemicals that create good feelings and energy along with group connections (Levitin, 2008).

Issues That Can Be Addressed in Different Phases

As phases progress, the group's thinking becomes clearer, and their moods become more hopeful, and Jennifer and other group members will be able to address more complex issues.

Changes in Discussion Level

As phases progress, group members will be able to talk more coherently and with more insight about their problems due to increased hope and clearer thinking. In phase one Jennifer and other members in the group are having difficulty finding words and putting their thoughts together well, so discussions may be shorter. Closure activities, such as a "blast-off" or "hand squeeze" that require less discussion may be useful.

Global Outcomes With Drama Therapy Interventions

As mentioned in Chapter Four, global outcomes involve complex skills and abilities that are components of mental health and which show up as deficits across many diagnoses in the DSM-5. Addressing these outcomes as treatment goals is often more difficult than addressing symptoms because of their complexity; however, taking the time to address global outcomes like emotional or behavioral regulation, sensory integration (SI), or locus of control (LOC) can improve many symptoms simultaneously. This requires thinking of participant needs from a wider perspective, as a whole functioning being, rather than as a list of negative symptoms that need to be fixed. Creativity, spontaneity, and LOC bring joy and empowerment into functioning. Strong executive functioning (EF) and SI make life tasks easier to accomplish.

Global Outcomes With Drama Therapy Interventions

Creativity

- Is there anything within the diagnosis that hinders creativity?
    - o If so, do you want to include a creativity treatment goal?
- Does your participant/group believe that they are creative?
- Does your participant/group feel afraid/unconfident in a specific art area?

Spontaneity

- How much spontaneity does your intervention require?
  - o Is there anything within the diagnosis that hinders spontaneity? If so, do you need to:
    - ■ Include a spontaneity treatment goal?
    - ■ Include teaching of spontaneity skills?

Sensory Integration (SI)

- If your participant has SI issues, what do you need to consider with regard to:
  - o Intervention materials
  - o Interventions themselves
  - o Included as part of the treatment plan

Metacognition

- Is your participant/group capable of metacognition? Populations such as people with IDD, dementia, and young children may have difficulty talking about the life-drama connection.
- Does your participant/group overintellectualize? Do they become easily overdistanced?
  - o If so, they may sound like they understand the life-drama connection and the emotions discussed, but in reality, they do not. You may want to consider emotional explorations versus metacognitive ones after the interventions are over.

Emotional and Behavioral Regulation

- If the participant/group are not able to regulate emotions and behaviors, could interventions trigger them to:
  - o Lose emotional control
  - o Lose behavioral control
  - o Dissociate
- If the participant/group are overregulated in terms of emotions and/or behaviors, could interventions trigger them to:
  - o Shut down emotionally
  - o Refuse to participate
- Does a treatment goal need to be added to help improve regulation?

Locus of Control (LOC)

- Does your intervention require a more internal or external LOC?
- Does your participant/group have a more internal or external LOC?
- Are there group dynamics that come into play if the LOC is widely different between group members, leading to a lack of understanding of each other's points of view?
  - A group could have a similar LOC due to past experiences or diagnoses.
  - A group could have a mix of LOCs.
  - One group member could be extremely internal or external in their LOC in comparison with the rest of the group.
- Do you want to incorporate changing your participant's/group's LOC as part of the treatment plan?

Creativity

Creative arts therapists believe that all humans are creative. Sometimes early in life or in school, people are told that they are not creative, so they will typically downplay their creative abilities. Group members who are depressed often do not feel creative. Jennifer and her group will probably struggle with belief in their creativity; they will need encouragement to take creative risks and need to be set up for success early in phase one.

Spontaneity

Initiation tends to be muted in participants who are depressed; this will negatively affect spontaneity. Many drama games used in warm-ups will enhance spontaneity. This will encourage Jennifer and others in the group to engage in spontaneous thoughts and actions. Spontaneity is infectious and can easily spread from one member of a group to another.

Sensory Integration

The "klutziness" often observed in people who are depressed is probably more a function of lack of awareness caused by impairment of EF rather than SI issues.

Metacognition

Metacognition tends to be impaired in people who are depressed. They overfocus on the negative and avoid the positive. In addition, because of rumination, decision-making skills are impaired. An external stressor, like the very real job discrimination Jennifer has experienced, naturally leads to sadness and rumination. Adding to that outside stressor, Jennifer's normal reactions have been funneled into a depressive cycle that she is stuck in. Jennifer's metacognitive abilities related to follow-through, decision-making, and initiation need to be reignited through drama therapy. Drama therapy interventions that involve role-play, such as sociodrama, developmental transformations, and role method, can help generate new perspectives and provide practice for approaching obstacles with renewed vigor.

The symptoms of depression and lack of sleep may hinder working memory, sequencing, focus, and attention span. Adaptations that may need to be considered include presenting information clearly, concisely, and at a little slower pace so Jennifer and the rest of the group can comprehend what is being said. Directions should be given one at a time, rather than in a long sequence. Jennifer is physically tired; however, physical activity can energize her and may balance her low affect. It may also make it easier for her to sleep at night.

Emotional and Behavioral Regulation

Jennifer's emotional and behavioral response to depression is to become overdistanced and shut down. She needs to reconnect her emotions with her body. Rather than just talk about her feelings, embodying them physically would help her find balance and begin to take action again. One way to do this could be to have her enrole group members to portray her emotions. She could speak with her emotions and then role reverse with them. Through a psychodramatic exercise like this, she would be able to move from concretization to observed modeling to embodied experience.

Locus of Control

Jennifer's current LOC score is on the external side. Research has shown that groups who are oppressed often have more external LOC (Nowicki, 2016). Jennifer's experience of discrimination at work has supported her feelings of not being in control, as have her religious beliefs. She can be encouraged to increase her role repertoire by taking on powerful, decisive types of roles. She can be encouraged to make assertive choices in scenes. In addition, dramatic activities in which she can engage in problem-solving individually or with a small group can demonstrate to her that she has agency.

Use of the Structure of Drama Therapy Session in Treatment

The structure of a drama therapy session creates a safe container for the work of the group. This structure is ritually the same each time the group meets, creating a dependable pattern that participants come to rely on. Elements of this ritual structure are the check-in, the warm-up, the main drama activity/intervention, and the closure.

Check-in

A check-in is a ritual go-around in which all members of the group, including the therapist, who usually starts, reports on how they are feeling at the moment. A check-in might require participants to say what emotion they are feeling or to find a metaphor to describe their current state. The therapist might ask, "If you were a color, what color would you be?" or "If you were an animal, what animal would you be and why?" This allows the therapist to take the "emotional temperature" of the individuals in the group and assess what kind of warm-up is needed. It also allows the group members to become aware of how others are feeling, who needs support, and who is able to provide support during the session.

Opening rituals for therapy also provide consistency for the group. They know what to expect and, as a result, feel safer. Rituals often reduce anxiety. This can be helpful for any group, but could be especially helpful for young children or individuals who need structure in their schedule, such as people with attention deficit hyperactivity disorder (ADHD), ASD, or obsessive-compulsive disorder (OCD). In a group in which participants are active and rowdy, an opening ritual can gather everyone's attention and calm everyone down. In a group like Jennifer's, which consists of people who are experiencing anxiety and depression, a ritual opening is like a gentle call to a safe space in which hearts can open and hope can be regenerated.

Check-ins

- Will your check-in work best if it is ritualized and the same each session, or will it work best if it is varied each time?
- Does your check-in need to be direct, or can it be metaphorical?
  - Can your group understand metaphor?
  - If not, can they learn to use metaphor?
- Does your check-in need to be embodied?
  - Can embodiment wait for warm-up?

Ritual Versus Varied Check-in

Jennifer and the group need to be challenged to expand their perspectives about themselves and their emotions; therefore, a variety of metaphorical check-ins might help provide insight or distance in thinking about their emotions. A ritual approach could provide stability and safety. Jennifer's group will be warming up each time with "the magic box." They will be encouraged to take any emotion that would get in their way of participating and put it in the "magic box." Different prompts can be used in this check-in to provide variety.

Direct Versus Metaphor

Jennifer's group can understand metaphor.

Embodiment Factor

The more embodiment used with Jennifer's group, the better. Hence, the choice of the "magic box" for check-in. It requires participants to reach for the box, open it, pantomime what they are taking out or putting in, closing it, and passing it to the next person in the circle.

Warm-up

The warm-up brings the group members together in the here and now. One of the primary purposes of warm-up is to build trust and form a therapeutic relationship. It focuses the group's attention on each other and the therapeutic work. It involves everyone in the group and encourages them to make eye contact and engage with each other. The warm-up is designed to move the group from being disembodied and unfocused to becoming embodied and focused. If there will be physical activities later in the group, a warm-up can loosen up the muscles of the participants, so they are ready to move. Sometimes the warm-up can introduce or support the theme of the main dramatic intervention for the session.

Each group or individual needs different amounts of warm-up in order to be ready to work. Sometimes, especially in the first phases, more warm-up is needed to get participants to open up and feel comfortable with each other and with drama therapy. There are times when the warm-up can become the intervention. For example, the game "tangling" (also known as "knots") can be used as a warm-up or can be used as an intervention. When a group enters the session and are appropriately psychologically distanced, usually less time needs to be spent on warming up than when they enter frustrated, angry, or sad.

Even if a group is highly motivated to work, a short warm-up brings everyone in the whole room together in the here and now. Much like therapists need to leave their baggage at the door when leading a group, the group members need to leave their baggage at the door so they can focus on therapeutic change. Because warm-ups provide a shift in focus and a sense of beginning, they mark the boundary between the regular world and the world in which change can happen.

When choosing a warm-up activity, be mindful of the diagnosis of the group and issues that individuals might have that could trigger unexpected reactions. For example, balloons are fun, but if your group has SI disorders or PTSD, a balloon breaking can be a problem. There are certain games, such as "bang!" or "murder" which could be contraindicated with troubled youth from violent neighborhoods, people who are grieving the loss of someone who has been murdered, or participants who have experienced war, rape, or other violent traumatic events.

Do not overlook the importance of warming up. A group can regress to an earlier phase of treatment or individuals can regress to the point where they refuse to participate if they are not warmed up. If the therapist experiences significant resistance to engagement in main drama therapy activities, it is helpful to evaluate if the participants had enough warm-up.

Warm-ups

- How much warm-up is needed?
- Does your intervention later in the session need a specific warm-up?
- Is the warm-up the intervention?
- What do you need to consider regarding diagnosis and individual factors?

Amount of Warm-up Needed

The members of Jennifer's group probably need about 20 minutes of warm-up in phase one as they are feeling isolated and disconnected. The physical lethargy of depression often requires more warm-up. They need to have fun.

Warm-up for Intervention

When preparing a group for psychodrama, a game in which participants switch roles might provide warm-up for role reversal, or for an intervention where listening is crucial to a successful outcome, warming up with the telephone might be helpful.

Warm-up as Intervention

Often in phase one participants make discoveries during the warm-up. When this occurs, the warm-up can lead directly into a therapeutic discussion. This may happen in sessions with Jennifer's group. A rousing game of the "winds are blowing" may generate physical and emotional changes. Bringing participants' awareness to these at the end of the game could develop into a discussion about ways to energize themselves and connect with others in their daily life.

Diagnosis and Individual Factor Considerations

Because the ability to initiate and other EF are not at their peak with depression, warm-ups involving the body will be imperative.

Main Drama Therapy Activity/Intervention

The main drama therapy intervention usually takes up most of the time in a session. If picked carefully, the check-in and warm-up can guide the participants directly to the main activity. However, in situations when participants arrive for group overdistanced or underdistanced, the preparation for the main activity might need to change to rebalance group members. Issues that are shared in these early parts of the session may reveal a crisis that needs to be dealt with immediately or a more relevant exploration that the group needs to undertake. The drama therapist must be flexible to the needs of the group.

Closure

Closure brings the session to an end. It sums up the work of the session and pulls together any loose ends. Participants are able to leave feeling calm, collected, and together. Deroling is a type of closure. Sometimes interventions that are highly emotional and engaging require deroling and closure before moving onto the next intervention.

Closure After an Intervention

Deroling
At the end of an intervention, like an improvisational scene, there may be a need for closure in the form of deroling. Deroling is the ritual disengagement from a

role that a participant has taken on during an intervention. At the end of the intervention, the participants are often left with the residual emotions and thoughts of the characters they were playing. Very emotional roles can be difficult to leave. Roles very close to one's own personality may also be difficult to leave. Deroling involves release of the role's cognitive, emotional, and physical aspects from the actor to enable a return to a neutral self.

The specific deroling technique used depends on the depth of the connection with the role (Bailey & Dickinson, 2016). Sometimes just shaking off the role is enough: releasing the muscular tension and posture of the character. At other times, a ritual is needed. If the actors were using props and/or costumes that represent the characters, taking them off and formally returning them to the group leader can help the actors take off the characters. The actor can say something like, "This scarf and crown don't belong to me; they belong to Queen Constance. I am not her; I am Lisa." The group leader then responds, "Thank you, Lisa. I will put these away. We can use them again in another scene," or "These are not yours; they belong to Queen Constance—you are Lisa, a member of the drama group" (Bailey & Dickinson, 2016).

Participants who are watching an intervention may also need to be deroled. A normal aspect of witnessing and empathy is mentally taking on the role of the characters and imagining what they are feeling as the scene progresses. Audience members typically identify with the protagonist of a scene or a psychodrama. The term for identifying with characters and participating imaginatively and empathetically in a story is called *narrative transportation* (Greene & Carpenter, 2011). The witnesses are imaginatively and emotionally transported into the scene and vicariously take on the roles and emotions. Witnesses may need to get up and shake off the character they have been identifying with or move around to a different spot in the room to break the spell of the scene.

Discussion

While the therapeutic goals of the role-play may have been for the participants to express themselves, discussing the ideas, emotions, and conflicts from the scene is important for processing the work and deroling from it. In discussion, the therapist can assess if something came up in the work that was unexpected and that now needs to be explored. Look for nonverbal behavior that indicates there is still emotional residue after deroling the actors and when the discussion starts to come to a close. Pay attention to actual behavior, such as difficulty letting the character go, disruptive behavior, a lot of side-talking about the role-play, or overly emotional responses (Bailey & Dickinson, 2016). These may mean more discussion and closure is necessary before moving on.

A discussion can be facilitated through a series of questions that move from close-ended to open-ended to closed-ended. Close-ended questions ask for a specific answer. Open-ended questions allow a variety of answers. The close-ended questions at the beginning should be leading and guiding questions about what the participants think in terms of the intervention. For example, "What emotions did you see expressed in the role-play?" "What conflicts did you see arise?" Open questions that follow allow for the life-drama connection, "What was it like expressing those emotions? What did you learn about yourself? Tell me more about that." Finally end with close-ended questions like, "Name three things that you learned from this intervention." Connections among ideas are made, insights sometimes appear, and the group can move on to the next intervention.

Closure at the End of the Group

Closure calms participants down and helps them transition to the next activity after drama therapy. Often it is used as a moment to reflect on what was done in the group that day and what was learned. It can also be utilized to close down any emotional issues that were explored which are still "in the room."

There are drama therapy approaches that do not process what has happened during the group. Typically, they end with a ritual in which the participant has a moment to end the therapeutic process for the day and to regroup before leaving. For example, at the end of a developmental transformations session, the drama therapy curtain is filled with any emotions or thoughts that the participant does not want to take home. Then it is "hummed" back up into the ceiling, and everyone is told to "Take a minute," before they leave (Johnson, 1991).

Some groups create closing rituals. For instance, a group might want to "pass the pulse" around the circle or chant a saying at the end of every session. At Second Genesis many groups were ended by singing "Lean on Me," which was the house song or by saying in unison, "Keep coming back! It works if you work it!"

An easy way to close is to ask participants, "What did you learn today?" or "What can you take with you from this session into the coming week?" This allows group members to reflect and make meaning of the work that has been done. A nonverbal, but embodied way to do this would be to create a sculpt around those same questions. A private verbal way would be to have each group member write for five to ten minutes in a journal before leaving. Journal writing can help develop intrapersonal intelligence (i.e., understanding the self and one's own emotions and thoughts).

It is important to leave enough time at the end of the group for wrapping up. If the main drama therapy intervention, deroling, and discussion takes longer than anticipated, leaving the drama therapist with only 3 to 5 minutes at the end of the session, it can be helpful to have a go-to wrap-up activity in your back pocket. Something as simple as a "blast-off" or "hand-squeeze" can be just the thing to end a group quickly and efficiently.

Closure for Interventions

- What type of closure is appropriate:
  - o Verbal processing
  - o Action
    - ▪ Ritual
- Have the participants who were involved in the intervention been deroled?
- Have the participants who were witnesses to the intervention been deroled?
- How much metacognition is needed in order to wrap up?

Closure for Group Session

- When does the session end? Is there enough time left to do the wrap-up that was planned, or does it need to be changed?
- What type of closure is appropriate:
  - o Verbal processing
  - o Action
    - ▪ Ritual
- Have the participants who were involved in the intervention been deroled?
- Have the participants who were witnesses to the intervention been deroled?
- How much metacognition is needed in order to wrap-up?

Type of Closure Needed

Jennifer's group is able to process verbally and through action. A concrete, physical wrap-up, which reviews what Jennifer and the group are taking away from the session, could be better than a verbal one in order to subvert the rumination that tends to go along with anxiety and depression. For example, while sitting in a circle, each person could say a word or phrase and take a pose that expresses their take-away for the day.

Conclusion

In the previous chapter the symptoms identified for Jennifer, our fictional participant, were linked to a DSM diagnosis along with the observable dysfunctions and global treatment outcomes. The specific cultural aspects that could be influencing Jennifer's experience were explored. From this, a treatment plan was created for Jennifer as she began drama therapy treatment in phase one.

In this chapter, the reader has been guided through the next part of the drama therapy decision tree with our fictional participant. This part of the decision tree looks at the phase of treatment the participant is in, the psychological distance of the participant and group, and the drama therapy pie in order to pick appropriate interventions. In addition, how these basic components interact with each other was explored. Further considerations were given to the overarching global outcomes: creativity, spontaneity, SI, metacognition, emotional and behavioral regulation, and LOC. Basic group structure in drama therapy which can also contribute to the decisions made by the drama therapist was discussed.

The drama therapy decision tree allows what often appears to be unconscious and intuitive knowledge to become a conscious framework available to drama therapists when planning and working with groups, individuals, and other professionals. It allows drama therapists to go into group and individual sessions with a roadmap, clear on the goals and objectives to be addressed. The drama therapy decision tree creates a common language for drama therapists to talk with each other about cases and helps them translate what they are doing into terms that traditional psychotherapists and other helping professionals can understand. The full drama therapy decision tree can be found in Appendix A.

6

A Systematic Method for Drama Therapy Treatment Evaluation

This chapter covers how to evaluate whether the drama therapy interventions are working to meet the objectives in the treatment plan. When objectives are not being met, interventions might need to be adjusted or revised. When objectives are met, new objectives and/or goals are added to the treatment plan so the participant can continue to make progress.

Susana Pendzik (2003, 2008, 2012) has created a drama therapy based evaluation called the *six-key model* which addresses the progress of treatment in drama therapy terms and can be translated into traditional clinical terms in addition to being used for assessment. The six-key model is able to show change in terms of individual objectives and within a more complex spectrum of outcomes, such as executive functions (EF), sensory integration (SI) or creativity. Each key will be explained with examples given of how a fictional participant might be assessed using them. To provide a variety of case examples, the six-key model will be demonstrated with Jarrod, a fictional participant who has a substance abuse diagnosis.

Susana Pendzik's Six-Key Model

Susana Pendzik, PhD, RDT, head of the drama therapy graduate program at Tel Hai Academic College in Israel, created the six-key model to provide a systematic way to talk clearly about the therapeutic interventions and outcomes of drama therapy using the language of theatre and drama therapy (2003). The six keys can assess how a participant progresses within a session and across sessions. As she says, "it can provide the therapist with much information about a person's inner world, interpersonal relationships, and ego functions" (Pendzik, 2012, p. 198). The model can also be used to look at the progression of a drama therapy group. Even though the six-key model is conceived in theatre and drama therapy terminology, it can be translated into the traditional psychological change language that the treatment team uses. When looked at over time, the six-key model can demonstrate how participants are moving (or not moving) through the psychotherapeutic process. When drama therapists understand these connections, they can communicate to their clinical team the work they are doing in a manner that the clinical team can understand. For those unfamiliar with the six-key model for assessment and intervention, each key will be described in the following paragraphs.

Key One: Passage—Entering and Exiting Dramatic Reality

This is the first key because this is where drama therapy begins—with the ability to go into dramatic reality, to use one's imagination, and pretend with self and others. Participants arrive at each session in ordinary reality and are invited by the therapist to enter dramatic reality through a game, scene, or other type of dramatic intervention. Once in dramatic reality, participants need to be able to come back to ordinary reality when the scene is ended. Participants need to know what is real, what is pretend, and not lose sight of either in the session.

The ability to go into dramatic reality is a human ability that typically is cultivated in childhood during the preoperational period. Imagination, a precursor to abstract thought, helps children explore ideas and possibilities that could become reality and allows them to begin thinking symbolically (Vygotsky, 1978). Traditional clinicians sometimes wonder if having certain participants (specifically, those with schizophrenia or dementia) entering dramatic reality would be dangerous because of their poor reality testing skills; however, entering into dramatic reality is a way to practice reality testing. For participants with schizophrenia or Alzheimer's disease the drama therapist can use concrete dramatic processes, such as focusing on role development, and concrete tools like costumes and props. In this way drama therapy can be an avenue to practice for those struggling with reality testing in a safe way.

Dramatic reality can help deal with the cognitive distortions related to reality testing that exist in many diagnoses, whether that is catastrophizing, overgeneralization, personalization, polarized thinking, minimizing, grandiosity, filtering, or control fallacies. Developing a character with a different perspective from the participant can lead to a willingness to entertain another way of looking at a situation or watching others try out different tactics to solve a problem in a scene. A participant who tends to have an external control fallacy could discover through scene work that he does have the ability to solve problems himself. A catastrophizer or minimizer could be put into a situation that is totally chaotic, such as dealing with an erupting volcano on an island. A catastrophizer could be required to develop a character who minimizes the problem, and a minimizer could be required to develop a character who catastrophizes.

If participants are unable to enter dramatic reality, it could be that they do not have enough developmental experience with play. This could be the result of early trauma, abuse, or neglect, or it could be through lack of opportunity to play caused by isolation. These kinds of participants need to learn how to play, and the drama therapist will have to become a coach in basic play and imagination skills.

Other participants might be unwilling to enter dramatic reality for other reasons. They might fear that they will lose themselves if they enter dramatic reality. Some participants could be afraid that they will reveal things about themselves that they do not want to share. They might fear that once they enter dramatic reality, they will not be able to control how the other participants behave toward them. Rather than needing to be taught play skills, an unwilling participant needs to feel safe and may need to be warmed up more than other participants in order to join the play willingly.

A therapist must be able to recognize the difference between the unable participant versus the unwilling participant. In traditional therapy, therapists are taught to address resistance, so the default mode is often to identify the participant as unwilling rather than unable. Keep in mind when using the first key to ascertain whether a hesitant participant has a deficit rather than an unwillingness to be involved.

A common mistake for an early career therapist is to push unwilling participants to jump into play too quickly or to move them into deeper therapeutic work too quickly. It is important not to try and force a participant or a group to move to a place for which they are not ready. In drama therapy more time can be spent in providing participants with practice in entering and exiting dramatic reality.

Key Two: The Quality or Style of Dramatic Reality

Once participants enter dramatic reality, the therapist will discover the quality of the participants' experience there. A participant may enter dramatic reality and become self-conscious or distracted, unable to focus on the character or role being played, and as a result leave dramatic reality before the end of the scene. Some participants may switch back and forth between dramatic reality and ordinary reality repeatedly during a scene to ask questions ("Am I doing this right?"), pay attention to someone watching ("Hey, don't laugh at me!"), or be otherwise distracted. This may be caused by an inability to sustain attention or because of self-consciousness and low self-esteem (the imaginary audience phenomenon/spotlight effect). Some participants may not be able to sustain the emotions created in dramatic reality and jump back out as soon as they begin to feel something. This could be from a lack of ability to regulate their emotions. Sometimes a participant is lacking in spontaneity or the willingness to follow the improvisational rule of "Yes, and ..." This can "gum up the works," and the scene can come to a screeching halt, taking all the participants in the scene out of dramatic reality. Experience in scene work, drama games, and other drama therapy interventions over time can develop these skills.

Another aspect of quality is for participants to be able to match each other's level of investment and belief in the drama. Rich dramatic reality will take participants deep into a scene. On the other hand, overinvestment can create a situation in which someone can get hurt. For instance, if a knight is battling a dragon and instead of pretending, actually hits the actor playing the dragon over the head with his prop sword, there can be blood and injury (which again takes everyone back into ordinary reality to deal with the emergency). The drama therapist often needs to teach stage combat skills and talk about stage conventions. Overinvestment can indicate where the physical and emotional boundaries of the participant lie. If overinvestment in scenes happens frequently, the participant's treatment plan may need an added goal relating to the development of healthy boundaries.

Another aspect of the quality of dramatic reality is how the participants use the space. The quality is high if participants are able to invest their bodies by really believing in the imaginary world, moving freely within the space, and using objects as if they are objects within the imaginary world. A participant, who just stands still with their arms glued to their sides, is not inhabiting the dramatic world, unless, of course, the character in the scene has been frozen in that position by an evil wizard. If there is a constant low level of commitment and motivation by a participant, it is important for the drama therapist to discern if this is a general deficit that needs to be addressed in treatment or a lack of buy-in to therapy.

Developing a strong quality in dramatic reality is not about aesthetic concerns as when someone is learning to be a good actor. The therapist should not give participants feedback the way a drama teacher or theatre director would. However, if a participant is deeply engaged in the dramatic reality, an extremely effective dramatic scene will often result. When participants are invested, the dramatic space becomes believable. If they create a willing suspension of disbelief for themselves, the other participants and the therapist will be able to suspend their disbelief as well.

Key Three: Roles and Characters

Pendzik differentiates between *roles* and *characters*. She sees roles as archetypes and characters as differentiated fictional individuals. She says, "The roles are the container for the personification of the character" (S. Pendzik, personal communication). For instance, mother, king, or warrior would be roles, while a loving, but exhausted mother of a large family, a wicked king who has stolen all the land from his subjects, and a victorious, brave warrior who is homesick for his wife would be characters.

The drama therapist looks at the types of roles and characters that a participant chooses to see if there is a pattern. For instance, if the participant is stuck playing victims in every scene or bullies other characters all the time, this would indicate that the participant has a very small role repertoire and might be stuck in one type of behavior in real life. A limited role repertoire does not only mean playing a specific character (like a doctor) again and again, it can mean taking on the same actions, attitudes, and emotions no matter what character is being played. Rigidity with personality traits is associated with a variety of diagnoses from autism spectrum disorders (ASD) to schizophrenia. The drama therapist can encourage the participant to take on other characters, behaviors, or points of view in order to practice more flexible behavior choices.

Expanding character choice can also be used to develop participants' empathy with others who are different. The ability to see other viewpoints than one's own is very functional behavior in ordinary reality, as is the ability to understand others' possible motivations. The more types of characters a participant plays, the more insight is developed into how other people might experience the world in a different way. Dr. T. D. Noble, a psychiatrist at Sheppard Pratt Institute, recognized in the 1930s that patients who participated in drama activities were better able to identify emotions in therapy sessions and were willing to experiment with a variety of new behaviors in their lives on the unit (as cited in Phillips, 1994). More recently, an undergraduate drama major at Kansas State University who was diagnosed with ASD told Sally that the acting classes he took helped him see other people as living beings rather than "objects there for my pleasure" (G. Bolding, personal communication, 2007).

Key Four: Content Patterns—Plots, Themes, Conflicts, and Symbols

In terms of the fourth key, the therapist is looking for patterns and choices made about themes, plots, and approaches to conflict. Paying attention to the content is important as it provides insight into the core issues that the participants are dealing with. When participant choices are repeatedly dysfunctional in this key, the therapist can challenge participants to allow themselves to experience different, healthier choices. A participant, who continually avoids addressing conflicts in scenes, is revealing a fear that needs to be dealt with. Through careful observation of how conflicts are being avoided, the therapist can see whether the weakness is in self-confidence, verbal skills, or discomfort in hurting others' feelings. A participant, who enters into conflict too quickly, may be revealing an inability to listen to others, a lack of conflict resolution skills, or a focus on self that disregards the needs of others.

While the fourth key reveals where the individual is getting stuck, it can also reveal, in terms of the group, where the group dynamic may be stuck. This becomes something that can be processed in ordinary reality or taken into consideration for the next session. If many scenes are chosen to be about adolescents and their parents, the group may be metaphorically signaling that it is ready to move on from an early stage (phase one or two) to the working stage (phase three). Through their dramatic themes, the participants may be demonstrating their need to have more independence. Another theme that can reoccur is the need to kill off the authority figure in a scene. This can also symbolize the group's need to move to a more independent phase (working or termination) through their symbolic killing the authority figure in the group: the therapist. However, sometimes the issue is not the therapist, but a different authority figure in the participants' lives.

Key Five: The Response to Dramatic Reality From the Outside

The fifth key often is found in ordinary reality as the group talks about what happened during the game or the scene that was just completed. "As a witness to dramatic reality, the audience is endowed with the power to legitimize the experience" (Pendzik, 2003, p. 95). If the therapist observes that participants do not seem to be engaged in dramatic reality while a scene is going on, participants genuinely responding in key five would show whether they actually are paying attention or not during the enactment. While they may not have had a fully developed role, character, or scene in the dramatic enactment, articulate involvement in key five means that therapeutic work did occur.

Most important is the ability of participants to respond to what they did while they were in dramatic reality. The ability to own the work that was done and meta-process it, so that it is no longer unconscious material, is crucial. If participants successfully address issues in dramatic reality, but are unable to recognize and process that work, the life-drama connection has not happened. In drama therapy, the therapist can assess whether the participant is really ready to change because they have not only demonstrated the behavior in a scene, but have also identified and reflected on it afterwards.

The fifth key can also highlight where there is a deficit in another key. A negative or delegitimizing response from the group during a discussion may indicate that the group has picked up a pattern in one of the other keys that is stuck or not moving in a therapeutic direction. The therapist is also within the audience, and it is the therapist's responsibility to note discrepancies in terms of what did or did not happen that the participant or the group missed, so that important areas that need to be addressed can be. This brings us to the sixth key.

Key Six: The Meta-Reality—the Unmanifested Subtext

Meta-reality encompasses transference, countertransference, unspoken dynamics and feelings: the elephant in the room, which everyone knows is there but actively ignores. Pendzik says, "meta-reality [is] like a parallel story that wanders about between both realities without finding a place to belong" (2003, p. 96). Meta-reality is not present in every scene or every drama therapy session, but when it is, it has a big impact. Sometimes when feelings or conflicts are not being played out in a scene, but exist subconsciously in the participant's life, the drama therapist will start experiencing transference in the form of feelings of confusion, anger, or sadness that cannot otherwise be accounted for (S. Pendzik, personal communication, 2019). The drama therapist has the responsibility of incorporating the meta-reality into the dramatic or ordinary reality by moving it out of the in-between space so that it can be acknowledged and voiced by the participants. Timing is an issue. If the therapist brings unconscious material to the surface before the participants are ready to deal with it, they most likely will deny it. It can also undo work that was previously done to create trust and move the participant forward. The participant can backpedal in fear or overreact in an unsafe way.

This key is one of the most difficult to decipher, especially when first starting to do assessments. The difficulty arises because sometimes the subtext/meta-reality is an aspect of the work, and sometimes it is not; sometimes it is there, and the therapist does not see it. Sometimes a therapist can project their own "stuff" onto participants' unspoken issues. The therapist needs to be clear-sighted and honest when making a determination about meta-reality. In the early development of a group, the therapist is often making a mental note and looking for evidence in subtext in the work that follows. Immediacy, addressing what might be unspoken in the group, is the best way of confirming or disconfirming the existence of the meta-reality. Through immediacy, the therapist is able to engage participants more deeply in work.

A Drama Therapy Treatment Plan for Jarrod

Jarrod is 23 and addicted to opioids. He started taking Oxycodone pain pills after an accident he had on a summer job between his first and second years of college and quickly became addicted. He mixed his opioids with binge drinking at his fraternity. This behavior led to poor grades and ultimately resulted in dropping out of college. His parents have finally gotten him into treatment for the first time. He has detoxed and joined the drama therapy group at his six-month residential treatment program. Jarrod would be diagnosed with severe opioid use disorder, in early remission 304.00 (6C43.21).[1]

For a participant with this diagnosis, the drama therapist might create an initial treatment plan like this:

Goal One: Participant will develop the skills to navigate social relationships appropriately.

> **Objective One:** Participant will learn listening skills.
> **Objective Two:** Participant will learn how to accurately reflect back what others have said to him.

Goal Two: Participant will develop empathy.

> **Objective One:** Participant will be able to accurately identify the emotions of others.
> **Objective Two:** Participant will be able to identify emotions accurately in himself.

Jarrod has been assigned to a drama therapy group that meets three times a week for an hour and a half. There are eleven members in the group in addition to Jarrod. The group consists of men and women who have addictions to a variety of substances. This is Jarrod's first time in treatment. Most of the group have been in treatment before.

Connecting the Six-Keys to Jarrod's Treatment Plan

We have created a set of six-keys for Jarrod, our fictional participant, from his behavior in a fictional drama therapy group. Jarrod volunteered to play a drug dealer in a scene in which members of the group were practicing how to handle meeting up with someone from whom they had bought drugs in their active addiction.

Key One: Passage

Participant was able to enter dramatic reality easily, but had some difficulty leaving at the end of the scene.

Key Two: Quality or Style

At times participant was hyper-involved in trying to convince the other actor to buy drugs from him, but when he was not the focus of the scene, he seemed to become disengaged.

Key Three: Characters and Roles

Drug dealer, very manipulative, very intense, driven, unwilling to take no for an answer.

Key Four: Content Patterns: Plots, Themes, and Conflict

Control, self-promotion, manipulation, kept scene focused on the selling and purchasing of drugs only. Participant is not yet able to truly give-and-take in a scene because he does not listen deeply to his scene partners.

Key Five: Response to Dramatic Reality From the Outside

Others said he played the role so well that they felt a little triggered. He took this as a compliment. Therapist suggested that if he had really listened to what the recovering addict said in the scene, his character might have made a different choice or had different thoughts. He argued that that would be unrealistic.

Key Six: Meta-Reality or the Unmanifested Subtext

Participant does not seem to be aware that he has not recognized he is powerless over opioids because he will only act out characters who are in control.

This focus on self, the need to be in control, and need to manipulate others continued in several additional scenes, creating a pattern. Jarrod's treatment plan can be compared with information gathered from the six-keys to see if any of the objectives have been met or are still in need of being met. If they have not been met, the six-keys will tell the drama therapist exactly what directions to give Jarrod in future scenes in order to work on those objectives. So that the reader does not have to refer back to the goals and objectives, they will be restated prior to the discussion of how each of the six-keys relates to them.

Goal One: Objective One. Participant Will Learn Listening Skills

Key one is not necessarily related to this particular objective. Key two, however, is very connected to it. While he is within dramatic reality, Jarrod needs to continue to be present with his fellow actors. When we are able to observe Jarrod staying present in the entire scene because he is interested and listening to everything in the dramatic realm, not just his part in it, the therapist will know that change is beginning. In clinical language, at that point he would be not responding to others from the ego-driven, self-focused perspective usually taken by an addict. To encourage continuation of the change, the therapist could use dramatic interventions in which Jarrod practices improvising a conversation in which he responds to and builds on what his scene partner says. This involves learning the improvisational skill of "Yes, and ..."

Related to key three, the therapist would want to see Jarrod increase his role repertoire (i.e., develop a broader sense of identity) to include characters who can really hear the words and meaning of the other actors in the scene. He was technically correct when he argued that realistically a manipulative drug dealer would not listen to a potential customer. Instead of continuing playing characters of this sort, Jarrod might be assigned a character, such as a detective, parent, or teacher, who genuinely wants to discover what the other character wants or needs, and whose job is to verbalize that want or need.

In terms of key four, the therapist would look for scenes in which Jarrod explores the consequences that result from dealing drugs or negative behaviors that he habitually enacts in real life. These kinds of themes would help Jarrod learn consequential and causal thinking. Learning this only through verbal discussion is difficult, especially for an addict who is good at manipulating language; experiencing it through practice makes it concrete.

In key five, the therapist would want to see if Jarrod can identify when he is listening and when he is not listening to his partners in the scenes. In addition, the therapist will be able to see if he begins listening to discussions with the group in ordinary reality. These skills relate directly to improved metacognition (self-awareness, specifically).

Goal One: Objective Two. Participant Will Learn How to Accurately Reflect Back What Others Have Said to Him

Key one can allow us to focus on whether Jarrod is having difficulty leaving dramatic reality because he is not listening to the other actors and understanding when a scene is coming to an end. At first, the drama therapist may have to end the scene by calling "Scene!" When this is necessary, Jarrod needs to identify why the scene was supposed to be over. When he can respond appropriately to those same indicators in later scenes, the drama therapist will know he is listening to the other actors. This involves the EF of shifting attention between self and other and between self and environment. Key two for objective two is similar to objective one. One of the benefits of drama therapy is that multiple objectives can be addressed with one intervention.

In terms of key three, when Jarrod can expand his role repertoire to include characters that can take in what other characters say to him and respond back appropriately, he will be showing change. For instance, he is playing a father in a scene and his teenage son says, "Dad, you don't understand!" An initial sign of change might be if Jarrod responded with, "Well, Son, tell me what I'm not getting," instead of his typical, "Yes, I do! You are the one who doesn't understand!" Another sign of change would be if the son said, "I want to make my own decisions!" and Jarrod responded with, "I know you feel all grown up and that you are able to take care of yourself, but I'm your father, and I worry about you," instead of, "You don't know enough to make your own decisions!" This change would demonstrate he had learned perspective shifting (seeing the scene from the point of view of the other character and incorporating that knowledge into the dialogue), another aspect of EF.

Key four deals with the content patterns in the themes and plot. The therapist will know change has happened when Jarrod volunteers for scenes with fewer themes that revolve around manipulation and control. If he begins really listening and responding to other characters in scenes, themes of cooperation, problem-solving, and teamwork will start emerging. The therapist may also notice increasing themes that involve caring for others and thinking of the needs of others before self. This may demonstrate the beginning of developing empathy (see goal two, objective one).

Responses (key five) might shift to other participants' response to Jarrod, reflecting that there is more give-and-take in the dialogue of a scene. In group processing after scenes, other participants might tell Jarrod that he has just given them good feedback or advice on a problem. The therapist would witness more, "Yes, ands ..." and fewer, "Yes, buts ..." in scenes and in discussions afterwards. This demonstrates flexibility and in terms of group dynamics demonstrates group cohesion. With less, "Yes, buts ..." Jarrod is making fewer excuses for himself and integrating his responsibility for his actions. He also may start to be able to take constructive criticism and reflect openly about his own process while acting the scene.

Goal Two: Objective One. Participant Will Be Able to Accurately Identify the Emotions of Others

Key one will probably not be a useful gauge for this objective unless Jarrod does not want to enter into dramatic reality because he feels uncomfortable acting with others who get in touch with their emotions. Getting into dramatic reality requires a capacity for intimacy. Holding back for this reason could indicate that

Jarrod is beginning to identify others' emotions and that makes him feel uneasy, lost, or out of control. This would lead the therapist to create an additional treatment objective for Jarrod to learn to sit with and experience others' emotions. Key one allows the therapist to assess Jarrod's ability to understand boundaries and emotional regulation.

Within key two, Jarrod would show change when his dialogue within a given scene is directly related to the emotional content of his scene partners. If another character was upset, Jarrod's character reaction might include comforting, supporting, or gently questioning. In addition, he would be able to match the emotional intensity of the other actors in the scene and make the transitions of emotion and subject matter along with his scene partners.

Related to key three, Jarrod would be increasing his empathic abilities if he increases his role repertoire by playing characters who are able to listen and respond appropriately to other characters in scenes, perhaps choosing to be the parent, teacher or therapist. In key four, he would be able to create and sustain scenes that involved themes of identifying others' emotions. For instance, in a scene between a drug counselor and an addict, as the counselor Jarrod would be able to identify what the addict character was expressing in the moment, rather than projecting onto that character what he might feel in a similar situation. This means that the scene would follow its logical course, rather than be hijacked by the counselor character's misreading of the addict character's emotions.

Jarrod's responses in processing after scenes (key five) would demonstrate change if he was able to verbally identify the emotions that other characters in scenes were expressing. Acting partners would be able to verify that in discussions. When Jarrod is watching a scene, he would be able to accurately identify the emotions expressed by the actors. In addition to verbal responses, the therapist would see appropriate body language and vocal responses while Jarrod watched a scene done by others. Connection to the characters and actions in a scene would be expressed through emotional responses, such as crying, groaning, or laughing at appropriate moments or through body language, such as leaning in to watch more closely. The sixth key was not active in these scenes on empathy.

Goal Two: Objective Two. Participant Will Be Able to Identify Emotions Accurately in Himself

Key one might be an issue if the scene requires an emotional commitment, and Jarrod does not like the experience of being in touch with his own emotions. He might avoid being in a scene because he wants to avoid dealing with his own feelings. Some participants run from feelings because they cannot identify them: the emotion is experienced like a big frightening blob that could swallow them up. Change would be indicated if Jarrod let himself enter and leave dramatic reality with ease, indicating an understanding of the difference between emotional flooding and emotional flexibility.

Key two: The quality or style of dramatic reality might be disturbed by the same issue discussed in key one. Instead of avoiding dramatic reality all together, the participant might skim the surface and avoid conflicts, as well as emotions, that would naturally be coming up for his character in the scene in response to the offers made by other characters. When the therapist sees Jarrod expressing a genuine emotion in a scene, he will be demonstrating congruence and acceptance of the feeling.

In relation to key three, Jarrod will demonstrate that he can identify his emotions if he is able to turn those two-dimensional "stock characters," such as the proverbial drug dealer or another kind of villain, into unique three-dimensional characters. Within a scene, Jarrod's character would be able to say what he is feeling. For example, in a scene in which his fiancé breaks up with him, Jarrod's character might say, "I'm shocked—I didn't expect this," and later in the scene his character might say, "I'm hurt that you don't love me anymore" or "I'm mad as hell—go away and leave me alone!" Progress is shown not only in reflecting on his character's emotions and feelings, but also in taking roles and counter role characters. For instance, maybe the abandoned lover is the counter role of the proverbial drug dealer.

Relative to key four, the content patterns of the scenes Jarrod enacts should reflect the therapeutic process by showing a dynamic, flexible array and transformation of contents. His repetitive and obsessive issues would not continue to come up. Instead of drug-related content, a variety of subject matter may emerge connected to purpose in life, career choices, and family issues. In the above-mentioned break-up scene, the action would focus on how abandoned or betrayed Jarrod's character felt, rather than on how expensive the engagement ring was and how many paychecks went into buying it. Jarrod's responses in key five would include identifying emotions that his character or he felt during a scene and identifying emotions he felt while watching a scene done by others. Key six does not appear to be active.

Using the Six-Key Model to Evaluate the Growth of a Drama Therapy Group

The six-key model can be applied to assessing the therapeutic growth of the drama therapy group as a whole, providing an outside measure for the therapist of when the group is ready to move to the next phase/stage. As you may remember, the group that Jarrod is in has 12 members, men and women, who have been in treatment previously. Four of the group members have been in a drama therapy group previously and found it to be useful and enjoyable. They have served as group leaders to encourage the others. The first phase quickly captured everyone's attention, because group members had fun and achieved insights about communication, trust problems, and the universality of their addiction experiences. They now come to groups open to working together. The therapist has been through the drama therapy decision tree and decided that because this is a six-month residential treatment center that creating a performance would not be optimum because it is an open group with changing members over time. While there might be time to work on individual self-revelatory pieces, process-oriented work is more congruent and a better fit for the 12-step treatment model.

When a group is open, there tends to be a core created by the process that keeps the group working together. A set of norms is developed that stays within the space no matter who is coming in and out of it. When a new person comes in, the norms and rules are already established, and it is clear to them how to fit into the structure. In drama therapy, this can be achieved because of the drama therapy rituals that are always followed, where the norms are experienced at an emotional level rather than only cognitively. Therefore, if a group member who has been there for six months leaves, the core does not leave with that individual even though they helped create the core. However, if there are a significant number of new members entering the group at the same time, maintaining the core becomes practically impossible because not enough of the core members are left to hold the established norms. In such cases, new members often want to establish their own group norms, requiring the whole group to reenter the initial phase of group development.

A Six-Key Model Assessment of a Group in the Middle of a Phase/Stage (Not Ready to Transition to a New Phase/Stage)

To demonstrate what an assessment of a group might look like, we will use the fictional drama therapy group that Jarrod is in. Currently, we will pretend they are in phase three: role-play (Emunah, 2020) /cohesiveness stage (Yalom & Leszcz, 2005). At the end of each group session, the drama therapist looks at the overall functioning of the group in relation to the six-keys to observe what is happening on the macro level of the group as opposed to the individual level. We will pretend that this group is in the beginning of this phase, still working through the obstacles it presents, and not get ready to transition to the next phase.

Key One: Passage

Newer group members still struggle to enter and exit dramatic reality. They are still experiencing the spotlight effect and worrying about what others in the group are thinking about them. Older members enter and exit dramatic reality more easily, unless they are not completely warmed up or preoccupied with other issues happening in their lives. They are able to exit dramatic reality unless the intensity of emotion in the scene has been high. When this happens, they are in need of a longer, more complex deroling process.

Key Two: Quality and Style

Group members are able to stay in scenes for longer periods of time than before, but can still become distracted. When this happens, they break the flow of the scene and the concentration of the other actors. The newer group members go in and out more frequently than the older members.

Key Three: Roles and Characters

Most of the group members feel most comfortable acting out characters that appear very different from themselves. They seem to still need the distance that fiction provides, and they enjoy "getting out of themselves," as feels like a welcome break from their current reality. A few actors who consistently play the roles of victim or controller in their actual lives revert to these actions, even if the characters they are playing have been designed to challenge them to behave differently.

Key Four: Content Patterns

Actors still seem hesitant to confront their peers constructively in scenes. Conflicts, when they do arise, tend to turn into shouting matches. Themes enacted: dealing with authority figures, rebelling, and striving to stay in control. In scenes, responsibility tends to be externalized to authority figures, and characters try to cut corners when given tasks to do by authority figures. Plots tend to be better developed, showing a clear beginning, middle, and end.

Key Five: Response

Most of the characters chosen to be played are fictional, but the group members are starting to recognize the life-drama connection between the issues and conflicts witnessed in the scenes, and the conflicts they have enacted. The therapist needs to address discrepancies in the appropriate behavior of the character in comparison with the real-life behavior of the actor. However, a few group members are picking up on the need and responsibility to do this and are able to do it in a respectful manner. Newer group members have difficulty accepting feedback. Of course, they love praise.

Key Six: Meta-Reality

Group members are unable to recognize their own subtext, but can see it when the therapist points it out. The therapist is still sensing some hostility in the air toward a few of the newer members and hostility from those members back to the group. More work is needed to address the need for group support and individual "buy-in" from the newer members.

Interpreting the Data in the Above Six-Key Group Assessment

This assessment is identifying that the group is still in phase three: role-play (Emunah, 2020) stage three: cohesiveness (Yalom & Leszcz, 2005). The clues the group is not ready to move on are:

Key One: Passage

Newer group members still struggle to enter and exit dramatic reality. This puts them more in phase two in terms of skill level. They will most likely catch up with the older members by modeling them.

Key Two: Quality and Style

The quality of dramatic reality can be poor when group members are distracted; however, this has been improving each week.

Key Three: Role and Characters

The actors continue to play the same types of characters using their old choices and behaviors.

Key Four: Content Patterns

Constructive confrontation is not happening in many scenes. Conflicts are being avoided, overblown, or dealt with in simplistic ways.

Key Five: Response

The life-drama connection of games and scenes is recognized, but group members are not yet able to confront each other on behavior discrepancy in a respectful manner.

Key Six: Meta-reality

The newer group members have not yet been fully accepted, and while they have said nothing about this or their own lack of "buy-in," there is an unspoken sense of distrust in the air.

A Six-Key Model Assessment of a Group Ready to Transition to a New Phase/Stage

This is an assessment of the fictional drama therapy group several weeks later by the fictional drama therapist. This assessment shows a group that has matured. They appear ready to transition to the next phase.

Key One: Passage

All group members have been able to enter and exit dramatic reality easily most of the time. On occasion, a member may have difficulty entering the scene if not completely warmed up, or they may have difficulty exiting the scene if the intensity of emotion in the scene has been high.

Key Two: Quality and Style

Most scenes have a fluid, solid feel to them. Group members stay focused on their actions and on the other characters. From time to time, they might get distracted if they want a prop that is not there: Instead of making it up as part of the scene or pantomiming, they stop to look around for something more realistic. This can break the flow of the scene and the concentration of the other actors.

Key Three: Roles and Characters

A few group members have been able to play characters who are closer to their real-life problems, but most group members tend to choose characters that appear distant from themselves. Of course, those characters tend to have similar conflicts as the actors, but they may still need the distance that fiction provides. Occasionally, actors, who had moved on from playing the roles of victim or controller to explore new roles, will go back to the old roles. This seems to happen on days when these particular actors report feeling frustrated or stuck.

Key Four: Content Patterns

Actors seem to be more willing to enter into conflicts and work through them to a constructive resolution instead of immediately taking the easy way out. A healthier pattern has developed in terms of the themes chosen to be enacted: taking responsibility, asking for help when it is needed, and letting go of people, places and things that cannot be controlled. Plots tend to be better developed, showing a clear beginning, middle, and end.

Key Five: Response

Even though most of the characters chosen to be played are fictional, the group members are able to recognize the life-drama connection between the issues and conflicts witnessed in the scenes, and the conflicts that they have enacted. Group members have started to understand that the actors are not the characters in the fictional scenes and can discuss the choices the characters made separately from the choices that the actors made. The therapist still needs to address discrepancies in the appropriate behavior of the character in comparison with the real-life behavior of the actor most of the time. However, a few group members are noticing the need and responsibility to do this and are able to do it in a respectful manner.

Key Six: Meta-Reality

Group members are able to recognize the subtext of the scenes they are witnessing (tone of voice, unspoken feelings, intentions behind actions), but are not yet able to recognize their own subtext. This means that the group members are able to point out to each other what subtext they are missing, and the therapist needs to do this less and less. The therapist is sensing an unspoken desire on the part of a number of group members to move into deeper work on personal issues.

Interpreting the Data in the Above Six-Key Group Assessment

This assessment identifies this drama therapy group might be coming to the end of their time in stage three and are ready for stage four: culminating enactment (Emunah, 2020) /working (Yalom & Leszcz, 2005). The clues that this group is ready to move onto the next phase are:

Key One: Passage

Participants are able to enter dramatic reality with ease.

Key Two: Quality and Style

Participants can stay in dramatic reality for the whole scene.

Key Three: Roles and Characters

Participants are able to play a variety of roles.

Key Four: Content Patterns

A healthier pattern has developed in terms of the themes, and plots now have a clear beginning, middle and end.

Key Five: Response

The group members are able to recognize the life-drama connection between the issues and conflicts witnessed in the scenes. Some members are addressing discrepancies in scenes during discussions with respect.

Key Six: Meta-Reality

Group members are able to recognize the subtext of the scenes they are witnessing. The therapist is sensing an unspoken desire on the part of a number of group members to move into deeper work on personal issues.

Conclusion

Susana Pendzik's six-key model provides a rich strengths-based assessment tool for identifying when treatment objectives have been achieved and assists the therapist in identifying which objectives need to be pursued next in order to reach the treatment goal. The example of how to create a treatment plan and assess work done in a drama therapy group with recovering addicts provides a model for how the progress of a specific participant's goals and objectives could be examined. The drama therapist would have a treatment plan completed in the same manner for all the individuals in the group and might track the group's development as a whole through an overarching set of six-keys after each session. This kind of assessment could indicate when a group was ready to move from one phase to the next and could also help the therapist pick interventions to try for the following session in order to build upon the work just done and move the group forward.

NOTE

1. 304.00 is the DSM-5 diagnostic code and 6C43.21is the ICD-11 severity code. Both codes are noted in the DSM-5 diagnoses.

SECTION 3

DIVERSITY AND ETHICAL CONSIDERATIONS

7

Diversity: Cultural Competence, Adaptations, and Accommodations

Chapter Eight will cover other ethical principles related to the choice of interventions. This chapter focuses on ensuring that diversity is respected and incorporated into practice. The North American Drama Therapy Association (NADTA) code of ethics, Principle 5a speaks to nondiscrimination and diversity (NADTA, 2019a). To supplement this short statement, the Guidelines on Cultural Response/ability in Training, Research, Practice, Supervision, Advocacy and Organizational Change (2015) were developed by the NADTA Cultural Humility, Equity, and Diversity Committee in consultation with the British Association of Dramatherapist's Equity and Diversity SubCommittee (BADTH, n.d.), the American Art Therapy Association (AATA, 2011), the American Psychological Association (APA, 2017), the Canadian Association for Music Therapy (CAMT, 1999), and Counselors for Social Justice (Ibrahim, Dinsmore, Estrada, & D'Andrea, 2011).

Awareness of diversity is important to all psychotherapists. All therapeutic practice focuses on the individual needs of the participant. These cannot be addressed without understanding who that person is within their entire cultural context. When thinking about diversity, most people focus on the cultural context alone; however, diversity also includes differences in ability, both cognitive and physical. Cultural issues and ability issues sometimes seem to be pitted against each other. In spite of this, both need to be addressed equally. This can be achieved through adaptations and accommodations.

People tend to use the words adaptation and accommodation interchangeably; however, the words have different meanings. *Adaptations* change an intervention so everyone can participate in the same way. To adapt the game "the winds are blowing" for a group including people who use wheelchairs and people who are fully mobile, spaces in the circle can be marked with a piece of tape on the floor instead of using chairs. This way mobile people and wheelchair users can move to any empty space in the circle. In a group of participants who speak a variety of languages, tone of voice and communication could be practiced using gibberish instead of using one common language. Then everyone is using a made-up nonsense language.

An *accommodation* adds something to aid the participant who would have difficulty with the activity without actually modifying the activity. This could be accomplished for the mixed mobility group by having an assistant push a wheelchair-user during a dance so that they are free to engage with other dancers face-to-face and dance with their upper bodies. In a mixed language group, an interpreter for each language could be provided. The activity would not change, and the individuals who needed help understanding the language would be accommodated.

Adaptations and accommodations are needed for all aspects of diversity. Cognitive and physical challenges need to be included along with cultural matters. To this end, Chapter Seven focuses first on matters of cultural competence, then transitions to challenges involved in differences in ability.

Cultural Competence

Knowing a person's personal pronouns or ethnicity are just the top layers of diversity. The complexity and interconnectedness of an individual's experience in all the layers of identity comprise the wholeness of that person. Most likely each participant has intersectionality with a number of cultures, including but not limited to socioeconomic status, ethnicity, nationality, age cohort, region of birth, religion, profession, diagnosis and/or disability, gender, gender identity, sexual orientation, physical attributes, health status, and state of displacement (e.g., people who are immigrants, refugees, or homeless). For instance, a participant could be a lesbian, African American, middle class, social worker, who struggles with post-traumatic stress disorder (PTSD). Another could be a straight, white, male, working class, Irish Catholic, prison guard from Chicago, who is clinically depressed.

Just as important, each participant will see the drama therapist from a cultural standpoint. Drama therapists must be aware of how they are being categorized, and, perhaps, stereotyped depending on how they appear to others. When someone hears the name Dr. Susan White, the impression could be that she is a cisgender, Caucasian woman who comes from a life of privilege and had her college education paid for by her wealthy parents. Dr. White may visually appear to be Caucasian. In reality, he is a transgender Puerto Rican who grew up in a lower socioeconomic Latinx inner-city neighborhood. Part of cultural competency is

Dr. White's understanding that even though he identifies as Hispanic and is transgender, his participants may be viewing him as a Caucasian female. If any of his participants are distrustful because of how they perceive him, they may not be able to form a good enough therapeutic relationship with him. The responsibility of the therapist is to work through difficulties that come up due to a perception or misperception of themselves. Their job is not to change the perception, as sometimes this cannot be done, but to be aware of the issues that are impacting the therapeutic relationship because of the perception.

Becoming culturally competent requires self-reflection. Practitioners must understand their own cultural influences, intersectionality, and biases. In addition, privilege needs to be acknowledged and addressed. Types of privilege include, but are not limited to, being white, middle or upper class, male, cisgender and heteronormative. There is also ability privilege. People in the disability community talk about those without disabilities as TABs: temporarily able-bodied. Everyone who has ability privilege is one accident or illness away from becoming disabled.

The decision tree can help remind the drama therapist not to make a judgment about a participant without asking questions. The decision tree questions about diversity issues remind the therapist to check into these aspects of identity and do more research. Our knowledge, no matter what our background is or how much we study other cultures, is going to be incomplete. Cultural competence is a lifelong learning process.

For example, one misnomer about participants from a nondominant culture is that they are coming to therapy to focus on issues caused by their culture: either they do not fit into their culture or they want to acculturate into the dominant culture. More often than not, neither of these are cogent. They are usually coming to therapy because their mental health issues are the same as everyone else's. Always ask participants what they want to work on; do not assume.

Another example is that a participant who is deaf is a member of the disability community. The correct way to refer to someone who has the audiological condition of not being able to hear is deaf (lowercase). However, when referring to an individual who is part of a group of deaf people who share a language and culture, use Deaf (uppercase). Barbara Kannapel, a Deaf sociolinguist, defines Deaf culture as "a set of learned behaviors of a group of people who are deaf and who have their own language (ASL), values, rules, and traditions" (Gallaudet University, 2015, para. 2). Do your deaf participants identify as members of the Deaf community? Some do, and some do not. Misidentifying a Deaf person as a member of the disability community can interfere with the therapist's ability to create a therapeutic relationship.

Questions to Ask Yourself about Cultural Competence

- What are my cultural biases and assumptions?
- Am I aware of how the privilege/power I hold impacts the therapeutic relationship?
- What assumptions am I making regarding the culture of my participant based on prior experience with a similar culture or a similar participant?
- What aspects of my participant's cultural background is most central or important to them?
- In concrete terms, what have I done to get to know the participant and better understand their perspective?
- Do I have any strong positive or negative feelings toward my participant?
    - How are those feelings impacting the therapeutic relationship?
- Am I aware of my participant's perceptions of me?
    - If so, what are they? If not, I need to ask.
    - How are those perceptions impacting the therapeutic relationship?
- Am I aware of all the intersectionality this participant has?
- In concrete terms, what am I doing to show respect for my participant?
- What am I doing that does not show respect for my participant?
- What are the cultural components of the drama therapy intervention?
    - Is there a conflict between the intervention and the participant?
    - Is there a conflict between the intervention and the participant's culture?
- Does the participant's culture make the participant vulnerable to specific dangers?
    - Prejudice from other community members or a hate group
    - Deportation
    - Other governmental or legal ramifications
        - Will a certain intervention heighten those dangers?

Cultural Humility

Cultural humility is an aspect of cultural competency, involving the understanding that every interaction needs to be "other-oriented." Because our participants are at the center of the therapeutic action, their values, opinions, and points of view need to be prioritized. Participants need to be able to define their own cultural identity based on what they find important. The participants' view of themselves in terms of their origins and intersectionality are more important than the therapist's knowledge of their cultures.

The culturally humble therapist approaches each project and each participant interaction with openness and awareness. Instead of relying on past knowledge, the therapist seeks cultural understanding directly from the participant. The personality qualities and practices of a culturally humble therapist were explored by Hook and colleagues (2013) and are identified as follows:

> On the intrapersonal dimension, humble individuals have an accurate view of self. On the interpersonal dimension, humble individuals are able to maintain an interpersonal stance that is other-oriented rather than self-focused, characterized by respect for others and a lack of superiority.
>
> (pp. 353–354)

The basic theatre skill of taking on a role can help a drama therapist practice cultural humility. Role-taking requires understanding others (character or actual person) well enough to take on their thoughts, feelings, and objectives and see the world through their perspective. Role reversal also helps develop cultural humility as it provides practice switching from one character's point of view to another's. Drama therapists should not take the openness, flexibility, and empathy these interventions offer for granted. Supervision is a great place to keep one's practice in these skills sharp. Continuing education also sharpens these skills.

Power Differential

Power differential is everywhere. Humans tend to create hierarchical structures that affect relationships between people and how they function within systems. At the current time, power differential is not explicitly included in the NADTA ethics code; it is minimally addressed under the guidelines for therapists regarding informed consent. Drama therapists need to realize that they are in a position of power over their participants. This is especially true for participants who are mandated to therapy by the court system. Thinking of oneself as a facilitator instead of as a leader or director can prepare the drama therapist to gracefully step aside and allow participants, when they are ready, to take on more responsibility for the work of the group. The power differential in a therapeutic situation becomes a problem when the therapist becomes rigid, unforgiving, or focused on the participants providing validation for the therapist. A treatment plan can be influenced by a power differential when therapists believe that only they know what is in the best interest of the group. When a therapist steps into role and interacts with participants as a character, conductor, director, double, or joker, the therapist needs to ask, "Who am I doing this for?" Are the choices made in the best interest of the participants, or are they driven by the agenda of the therapist ("I know best." or "I can do this better.")? Ask yourself, "Is this a situation I absolutely need to step into?"

Inherent within drama therapy interventions are techniques to escalate or de-escalate the power differential. The foundation of improvisation ("Yes, and ...") puts all participants on an equal playing field. Participating in a game as a player as opposed to as the leader allows the power differential to be de-escalated. When the therapist has a participant step out of a scene and direct it, the therapist is sharing the power. The beauty of drama therapy is that power differential can be played with, as opposed to it being an elephant in the room that no one is willing to address.

Adaptations and Accommodations

Drama therapists need to ask questions with regard to diagnostic categories. Often adaptations or accommodations are needed to remove barriers created by specific diagnostic symptoms. Here are some questions to help pinpoint changes that might need to be made in activities, discussions, or other interventions.

Adaptations and Accommodations

Are there cultural adaptations that need to be made to drama therapy interventions?

- What is the native language of the participant?
  - o If it is not the dominant language the group is being conducted in, how well does the participant comprehend that language?
  - o Does the participant need a translator?
  - o Could the language barrier be addressed through:
    - ■ Simpler words
    - ■ More use of gestures
    - ■ Intervention adaptation or accommodation.
- Is there a change that would make the intervention more culturally relevant?
- If cultural appropriation could be an issue with a participant or participant group, what can be done to change it?

Are there adaptations that need to be made to interventions because of the diagnosis or an ability issue?

- Is the participant functionally mobile?
  - o If there is a mobility impairment, what assistance is needed?
    - ■ Gross motor functioning

        - Ability to walk
        - Ability to sit and stand
        - Ability to make large arm or leg movements
        - Coordination/balance
        - Fine motor functioning
        - Gripping/holding
        - Writing/painting
        - Use of tools or machinery.
    - Does the participant use a mobility device? If so, what adaptation is needed for interventions?
    - Does the mobility device itself impose limitations?
    - Does the mobility device create safety issues?
- Does the participant have a vision impairment?
- Is the participant deaf or hard of hearing?
- Does the participant have a medical diagnosis that could impact the group or session?
- Are any participants survivors of trauma?
- Are there cognitive adaptations that need to be made to drama therapy interventions because of the diagnosis or an identified disability?
    - Can the participant read?
    - Is the participant able to think abstractly or are visual and/or concrete materials necessary to clarify instructions?
    - Does the participant have normal working memory?
    - Can the participant keep sequences in order?
    - Can the participant focus/attend, or is the participant easily distracted?
    - What is the participant's reality testing?
    - Does your participant have organized or disorganized thinking processes?
    - What is the language comprehension of the participant? Will you need to use:
        - Simpler sentences
        - Simpler words
        - Avoid idioms.

Other adaptation or accommodations to consider

- Is the intervention age/ability appropriate?
- Is there a service animal that needs to be incorporated into therapy?
    - Service animal
    - Therapy animal
    - Animal assisted therapy
    - Emotional support animal.

Cultural Adaptations

Adaptations may be needed in a drama therapy group for language challenges, cultural relevance, or to avoid cultural appropriation. Assessing the need for cultural adaptations is continuous throughout the therapeutic process. Check with participants to make sure that the adaptation put in place eases challenges and removes barriers instead of exacerbating them.

Language Challenges

While drama therapy has many active, nonverbal aspects, words are needed for instructions, interventions, and discussions. Participants with language comprehension issues will quickly feel frustrated. Obviously, language challenges are present for second-language learners, but they can also be due to the use of unfamiliar colloquialisms or difficulty in understanding the dialects of regional communities.

If English is not the first language of group members, but the group is being conducted in English, everyone's level of speaking and listening comprehension is going to be a little bit different. The therapist needs to check with participants to make sure that what is being said makes sense. The difficulty could be with the speed of speaking, choice of words, complicated phrasing, or the amount of information being presented at one time. When one is learning a new language, it takes time to take in the words, translate them into your first language, and make sense of the meaning. This speeds up with practice, but no group will have all the members translating and making meaning at the same speed. Make sure that language is appropriate for the lowest level of understanding in the room. This does not mean to use language or a tone of voice that could be experienced as infantilizing or condescending. The goal is inclusion.

The opposite situation can be in effect. A therapist could be speaking the native language of the participants and not be a native speaker. Group members often appreciate this, and they are forgiving when mistakes are made. Even so, this will be problematic if concepts are misunderstood. The therapist needs to check with the group members frequently to make sure they understand what is being said.

When a therapist is working with participants from a different culture, different region, or a different age cohort, there may be words or phrases that are unfamiliar to the therapist or the group. The appropriate response is to say, "I don't know that term. What does it mean?" early on, rather than pretend for six months that the meaning is clear. Be aware if it is appropriate to adopt colloquialisms or slang used by the group. For example, if a white male therapist uses the word "bro'" when addressing African American male group members, they could feel that the therapist was appropriating their language. On the other hand, using "bro' " with a particular group may create an egalitarian connection that is appreciated. Always check with the participants.

Other accommodations could include the use of visuals, gestures, demonstrations and other concrete means to help improve communication in addition to translation. One of the strengths of drama therapy is the ability to incorporate a variety of modes of communication. If there are language challenges that cannot be accommodated in the group, it may be necessary to refer a participant to another group.

Making an Intervention More Culturally Relevant

There are various ways to make an intervention more culturally relevant to participants from diverse backgrounds. One way is to use art, media, stories, and other materials that are culturally specific as group members are already accustomed to using them. Fairy tales and folktales have versions specific to cultures all around the world. If the drama therapist were working with a group from a specific culture, it would seem more appropriate to use the version that the participants are familiar with. For example, there are 58 different versions of the tale we know as "Little Red Riding Hood" with 72 different plot variables that were written down between the first century and the current one (Nuwer, 2013; Tehrani, 2013). At the same time, the therapist should be aware of the specific symbolic and cultural meanings the tale has in its culture of origin.

A group from a collectivist culture might feel more comfortable with certain types of interventions over others. For instance, instead of psychodrama, which focuses on one individual in the group, the therapist could use sociodrama, which explores the shared central concern of the whole group. This would avoid putting one person on the spot to share personal details that might be culturally inappropriate to share. Both psychodrama and sociodrama use exactly the same techniques, but they focus on different ways of investigating social behavior.

Role method (Landy, 1991, 1993, 2009) is based on a study of theatrical roles found within Western dramatic literature. Roles in Asian and African drama were not explored as part of the taxonomy. When working with participants from those cultures, a therapist might need to be open to exploring roles beyond the Western canon. More importantly, they need to look at the roles that are chosen through the lens of the participant. One place to start might be to have participants create their own role inventory.

Typically, in the United States, puppets are seen as toys for children. This is not so in Asia and Europe, where puppets are an adult art form as well. Puppets are wonderful distancing devices and can be employed to help children and adults work through issues of trauma and shame. Making puppets from scratch allows participants to personalize and be in control artistically of their creation.

Rituals that are brought into drama therapy can give support and comfort to groups. Some cultures may feel more comfortable participating in rituals than others and therefore may be more open to creating and incorporating them. However, the therapist needs to be aware of the meanings rituals hold in specific cultures to make sure that the ritual is used appropriately. The therapist may need to think about rituals beyond the classic opening and closing drama therapy rituals in order to be more culturally inclusive and relevant to specific drama therapy groups.

Cultural Appropriation

Drama therapy is inherently multicultural in that there are theatre traditions and storytelling traditions in all cultures. When drama therapy incorporates multicultural traditions with cultural humility, interventions can bring comfort, support, and the experience of feeling understood to participants. Theatre artists make no secret of their propensity to steal good artistic ideas from others to use or adapt into their own works of art. This practice is so frequent that the artistic world calls it *influence* rather than *appropriation*. Because of this natural tendency to borrow, drama therapists need to be aware that when they freely adapt ideas to create new interventions, they may be viewed as culturally offensive or inappropriate.

Masks are theatrical and ritual artifacts in all cultures. Mask making is often used in drama therapy to assist participants explore identity issues. When participants create their own masks, there is less chance of cultural misuse because the work is focused on that person's therapeutic process. However, the use of masks becomes cultural appropriation when a drama therapist takes masks that are used in actual rituals, religious rites, or ceremonies and uses them in group improvisation or performance. This disrespects the original purpose of those masks and can significantly impact the therapeutic process, even if there is not a participant from the culture of origin.

The same goes for the use of musical instruments from different cultures. Sally inherited a very interesting looking percussion instrument from her grandmother's collection of musical instruments. It was included with the rhythm instruments for the improvisational musician in a class on playback theatre. After class, one of her Korean students told her very gently that it was an instrument used only in funerals in Korea. Needless to say, she took it home and has not used it since.

Cultural appropriation needs to be considered with each intervention. In the context of this book, there is no way to address all the areas in which drama therapists may find themselves culturally appropriating symbols, rituals, and artifacts into their practice; however, here is a checklist of questions to ask yourself about cultural appropriation. If you feel uncomfortable as you answer any of these questions or begin to doubt your motives in using a particular intervention, you should probably reevaluate using it.

Checklist to Ask Yourself About Cultural Appropriation

- Is my practice or artifact from the dominant culture?
  - If not, to which ethnic/racial/cultural group does the practice or artifact belong?
- Is the group that the practice or artifact belongs to oppressed?
  - If yes, does my use of the practice or artifact continue the oppression?
    - Does the practice or artifact represent the oppression?
    - Does the practice or artifact represent defiance of the oppression?
- Apart from any clinical benefit to my participants, how do I benefit as the therapist from using this practice or artifact?
  - By making money from selling it
  - By being seen as "cool" or "with it"
  - By being seen as "cutting edge"
- Why might my use of this practice or artifact make someone from the ethnic, racial or cultural group of origin uncomfortable?
- How did I learn about this practice, tradition, or material?
  - Did I find this on the Internet?
  - Did I read about it in a book?
  - Did I learn this in a training or class?
    - If I did, was it assessed by the presenter for cultural appropriation?
  - Did I learn this from practitioners from the culture of origin?
    - Did they give me permission to use it?
    - Were there any restrictions or guidelines?
- How am I honoring and giving credit to the group that created this practice or artifact?
- Am I modifying the practice or artifact?
  - How am I modifying it?
  - Why am I modifying it?
  - What legitimizes my changing it?
  - Am I explaining this to my participants?

Being culturally aware and having a sense of cultural humility takes a deep level of honesty, integrity, and willingness to admit error or lack of knowledge. Looking deeply into one's self and standing in one's integrity takes a tremendous amount of thought and energy. Often therapists want to be culturally competent;

they just do not have the desire, time, or the energy to put in the amount of work that is necessary to achieve competence. Privilege often misleads therapists who are members of the dominant culture to think they have done enough.

Often, therapists are so overworked that self-care goes out the window, leading to a state of apathy. When that happens, cultural competency joins self-care at the bottom of the to-do list. The harsh reality is that none of these are excuses. The commitment to cultural competence must be made and followed through on.

Adaptations and Accommodations for Diagnosis and Ability Issues

Mobility Functioning

Gross Motor Functioning

Gross motor skills involve large muscles of the body used for walking, sitting, standing, and other large body movements. Participants with limited gross motor skills may need assistance in interventions involving movement, but may have no difficulty creating dialogue, improvising a scene, or participating in discussions. If coordination is difficult for a participant, make sure that the movements required for an intervention are clear for safety reasons and to avoid potential embarrassment. Balance issues could cause a participant to become totally focused on self-stabilization and not able to attend to the therapeutic aspects of the intervention. Embodiment does not necessarily require gross motor movement and coordination: many embodied activities like sculpture, sandtray, and puppetry can be done without the use of gross motor skills.

Fine Motor Functioning

Fine motor skills involve small muscles in the hands, face, and feet. Participants with limited fine motor skills might have difficulty gripping a pencil or paintbrush, cutting with scissors, or doing other activities involving small, intricate movements. Many adaptive devices have been created to help with these problems and can be found through educational and therapeutic product companies. Grippers can be put on pencils or paintbrushes. Adaptive scissors can cut paper. Big rings that are easy to grasp can be put at the end of scarves or ribbons. Books, scripts or papers can be held in place by music stands or book holders.

Is the Participant Functionally Mobile?

A great variety of devices exist to provide people with mobility: wheelchairs, scooters, walkers, crutches, and more. People who use wheelchairs are not necessarily paralyzed. Some are able to walk short distances and only need a chair for long distance transportation. Some who use mobility devices may have electric controls that allow them to move themselves. Others may have wheelchairs that are moved manually. Ask your participants. They deal with their mobility device every day and will have ideas about what could work. It is not rude to ask.

When a group member uses a wheelchair or another large mobility device, the drama therapist needs to evaluate the physical space in which the group is going to be held. The Americans with Disabilities Act (1990) requires public accommodations be made accessible for people who have mobility issues. A few items to think about:

- The mobility device needs to access the building and the therapy space or theatre.
- Doorways need to be a minimum of 32 inches wide.
- Tables need a 30-inch clearance from the floor to the bottom of the table.
- Ramps need a minimum width of 36 inches with a railing or lip at the sides to prevent mobility devices from rolling off.
- Ramps need to have a slope of no more than 8.3 percent (for every 12 feet in length, the ramp should rise one foot in height).

For more information see *The Arts and Humanities Accessibility Checklist* (2013) and *Design for Accessibility: A Cultural Administrator's Handbook* (2005) available for free download at the National Endowment for the Arts website.

Blindness

Terms for difficulty in seeing include *partially-sighted*, *low vision*, and *legally blind* as well as *vision impairment*. Legally blind does not necessarily mean one cannot see anything. It means that vision is less than 20/200 in the better eye even with corrective lenses. The 20 in the ratio refers to how close to an object the legally blind person must be to see it in detail, and the 200 refers to how close to an object an average person must be to see the same amount of detail.

Depending on the specific condition, sight is affected in different ways. Each condition affects individuals differently, and accommodations will therefore need to be different. The therapy space should not have clutter or items on the floor that are easily tripped over. Some people use a cane to get around. The cane becomes an extension of the person, allowing them to "feel" when the texture or level of the ground changes. Some people have guide dogs (more on service dogs later in the chapter). There are people who may want someone guiding them from place to place. The guide stands beside the person, and the person gently touches the guide's elbow. The person will take movement cues from the guide's body (Bailey, 2010).

Not everyone who has vision impairments knows how to read Braille. Only 5% to 10% of people who are blind learn Braille (as cited in Bailey, 2010). There are many accommodations available through technology. Print materials from books to newspapers are available in audio format. In theatre and television, audio description services are available to describe the nonverbal aspects of the action, so the person with vision impairment can understand what is happening. Electronic materials can be made accessible on computers; Word has a read aloud feature on Review, and other audio tools exist. Hard copy materials can be enlarged before being printed by changing the font size on a computer or after by enlarging it on a copier. There are also many kinds of magnifying tools. Ask participants how best to create an accommodation for them; they will be able to suggest the cheapest and easiest way to do it for them.

In each session, let the person with the visual impairment know who is in the group by naming the participants when you speak to them and by having them identify themselves when speaking. Clue group members into doing this to make inclusion a fully welcoming experience. The therapist needs to verbally describe instructions clearly when someone with a vision impairment is in the group. Pantomiming actions and providing visual demonstrations will not be useful. Remember to verbalize "yes," "no," and all nonverbal communication. Remind other group members to do this, too.

The spatial awareness of individuals with vision impairments is very acute. It is possible for a person to memorize where all the furniture is in a room or on a set as long as those pieces are always in the same place. There are individuals whose sound localization abilities are so finely tuned that they can throw a ball directly to a person in a circle after hearing that person speak. Do not underestimate their abilities of being able to play certain games. If participants are willing to experiment, it is possible to explore new skills or accommodations in a fun, nonthreatening way. You and your group members may discover new strengths.

Most people who have vision impairments are very independent people. As familiarity with the space and with the others in the group grows, the accommodations needed for your participant with vision impairment may shift. Keep checking in with them so that their apparent confidence does not lead you to ignore their needs or continue to offer more support than they really need.

Deaf or Hard of Hearing

The hearing abilities of deaf and hard of hearing people range across a continuum from small losses to complete loss. Just as few people are totally blind, few people are totally deaf. Some use assistive hearing devices, ranging from hearing aids to cochlear implants. Today's hearing aids are so small that often no one except the user knows they are there. Cochlear implants have internal and external components. The implant itself is within the head in the ear, and a small microphone and transmitter are placed outside the head just behind the ear. They look a little like the old visible hearing aids.

The National Association of the Deaf Law and Advocacy Center (2003) have defined the cultural and linguistically competent mental health provider as someone who is able to communicate directly in American Sign Language (ASL). They should be deeply aware of Deaf culture and the linguistic differences it has from hearing culture, as well as the psychosocial impact of living with hearing loss in a hearing culture. They should understand assistive devices and services and know how to use them appropriately. If the mental health provider can use other sign and visual communication systems, that is a plus.

A variety of communication styles exist from lipreading only to cued speech to sign language. If a participant uses only lipreading, therapists must be sure to stand where their lips can be clearly seen. Other group members will need to be reminded to face the participant when speaking. Please note that even the best lip-readers miss significant amounts of communication, and it is rarely recommended for important communications such as therapy.

Cued speech is a visual system of communication that in English uses eight hand shapes in four different positions beside the mouth to indicate the phonemes being created. In spoken language, there are certain sounds that look identical. For instance, the *p* and the *b* sound different, but look the same. The hand shapes help clarify which sound is being made. Cued speech is more quickly learned than sign language. It has been adapted to more than 50 languages (National Cued Speech Organization, n.d.). Cued speech has grown in popularity since the invention of cochlear implants in order to clarify incomplete or distorted sound; however, it is not commonplace to use within the Deaf community.

Both cochlear implants and cued speech are controversial accommodations in the Deaf community. Research has shown that in order to learn how to hear through the implant and learn to speak, it is better to stop using ASL. From the Deaf perspective, individuals with cochlear implants are being taken away from the Deaf community and being integrated into the hearing community. Parents usually make the decision regarding cochlear implant surgery for their infant or young child. This takes the decision whether to be Deaf or not away from the child. The medical community sees cochlear implants as a cure for deafness, underlining their belief that being deaf is a disability. However, an implant is technically not a cure; it is a prosthetic substitute that stimulates the cochlea (Hearing Link, n.d.; Kilgore, 2019).

> The official position on cochlear implants from the National Association of the Deaf is: Cochlear implantation is a technology that is to be used as tool [*sic*] for some forms of communication, not a cure for deafness. Cochlear implants provide sensitive hearing, but do not, by themselves, impart the ability to understand spoken language through listening alone. In addition, they do not guarantee the

> development of cognition or reduce the benefit of emphasis on parallel visual language and literacy development. The NAD recognizes the rights of parents to make informed choices for their deaf and hard of hearing children, respects their choice to use cochlear implants and all other assistive devices, and strongly supports the development of the child and of language and literacy.
>
> (NAD, 2019a, paras. 2–3)

Deaf participants who are reimbursed for therapy through insurance can go to the insurance company to ask for a referral for a therapist who is fluent in ASL or for an ASL translator. Any publicly funded, for profit, or nonprofit agency is required by the Americans with Disabilities Act (1990) to supply a translator. The exception to this is if an undue burden would be placed on the business by supplying the accommodation. The undue burden exception is looked at on a case-by-case basis (NAD, 2019b). When using a translator, the hearing person (therapist or other group members) should look and speak directly to the Deaf person and not to the translator.

If the therapist places an emphasis on interventions with movement, pantomime, and physical expressiveness, Deaf participants' strengths will come to the fore and can be built on. Many Deaf people have excellent rhythm and enjoy dancing. Rhythm is understood not through their ears, but through feeling vibrations and watching movements. There is a famous Deaf drummer, Eveline Glennie, who says she taught herself to hear with other parts of her body (Glennie, 2003). This is a wonderful explanation of how the sensory experience of drama therapy can be experienced by individuals with hearing loss.

The following is a checklist of areas to consider in terms of accommodations. When working with student-aged participants, ask for a copy of their individual education plan (IEP). This will also provide helpful information regarding accommodations. The following website also provides resources for working with those who have hearing loss: https://successforkidswithhearingloss.com.

Accommodations and Adaptations Checklist for Participants With Hearing Loss

- **Communication and Instruction Accommodations**
  - o Obtain participants attention before speaking
  - o Frequently check for understanding
  - o Repeat and rephrase information

- Enhance speech/lip reading conditions (keep hands away from mouth, no gum, etc.)
- Clearly enunciate and allow extra time for processing information
- Use visual aids
- Present information in a simple, structured and sequential manner
- Provide handouts with basic information/outline for the session.

- **Physical Environment Accommodations**
  - Reduce auditory and visual distractions (carpet, sound dampening materials, reduced sound of AC units, etc.)
  - Bright lights
  - Room set-up to allow for everyone to be facing each other
  - Visual alarm systems.
- **Intervention Adaptations**
  - Break up instructions, step-by-step
  - Give many breaks during session (listening with a cochlear implant, lipreading, etc. is exhausting)
  - Provide supplemental materials
  - Have a partner/buddy system
  - Add other sensory components to a traditionally verbal intervention.

Adapted from Johnson, Benson and Seaton (1997) The IEP Checklist

Medical Concerns and Complications

Anytime a participant has significant medical issues, it is important to understand which symptoms, behaviors, or needs must be addressed during a session. There is a difference between having supplies available in the therapy space versus intervening in a medical issue. For example, before someone with diabetes goes into diabetic shock, their blood sugar drops. The symptoms of this include dizziness, shakiness, sweating, and nervousness. If they go into insulin shock, they will move as if drunk, displaying confusion and poor coordination. They may trip and fall or exhibit muscle tremors. When you know you have a person who has diabetes in a group, fruit juice or hard candies should be kept in the therapy space and made available if you see the symptoms of diabetic or insulin shock.

A drama therapist also needs to know if there are any medical interventions that need to be undertaken on behalf of a participant. Someone who has epilepsy might have a vagus nerve stimulator (VNS) that controls seizures when or just before they start to have a seizure. The VNS is implanted underneath the skin, usually just left of the chest area. A magnetic device carried by the person is swiped over the VNS when the person senses a seizure coming on. If the seizure starts, and the person has not swiped, the drama therapist should know where the magnet is and swipe for the person. During a tonic-clonic seizure the person is unconscious (hence the necessity of someone else stepping in to swipe the magnet). There is a specific way to swipe, so a lesson on what to do is necessary, because if the magnet is held over the VNS instead of swiped, the VNS will turn off (Shafer & Dean, 2018).

If a medical issue arises during a session, think before acting: Is the emergency more than a matter of basic first aid? If you have not been trained to medically intervene, do not! Phone for help. There are some interventions a layperson is not expected or qualified to take on. If a participant needs medications, such as acetaminophen, ibuprofen or aspirin, do not physically give it to them; the participant may take it, but the therapist may not dispense it. You may help if you have received training in advanced methods such as CPR (Cardiopulmonary Respiration) or AED (Automated External Defibrillator), but if you have not, and you make a mistake, you could be sued.

Here are a few common items all therapy rooms should have on hand:

- A basic first aid kit with gauze, Band-Aids, latex-free gloves, scissors, tweezers, and alcohol swabs.
- In case of bad nosebleeds, tissues will need to be on hand.
- In case of peanut allergies, the room will need to be sanitized before the participant comes in.
- In case of seizures, be sure to have a pillow available to put under the person's head.
- In case of latex allergies, have non-latex gloves on hand and check for latex in other supplies that might be used, such as balloons.

Have a place in your informed consent form where the participant can write down any allergies or medical issues you need to be aware of. Make sure you have emergency contact information for doctors as well as a family member to call. It is also important to know how to appropriately clean up any bodily fluids (blood, vomit, urine, etc.) if there is a chance a participant has hepatitis, HIV, or another pathogen.

Trauma Complications

For the purpose of this book, *trauma* will be defined in a broader context than the diagnosis of PTSD, because participants can present with a wide variety of reactions to past experiences. The therapist needs to know how to deal with those reactions appropriately. The DSM-5 defines trauma as resulting from an event in which an individual has had direct exposure to actual or threatened death, actual or threatened serious injury, or actual or threatened sexual violence (2013, p. 271). There are a variety of ways to experience trauma: direct experience, direct witness of a traumatic event, indirect experience (the trauma happened to a close family member or friend), or repeatedly seeing or hearing secondary details of trauma (as a therapist or a first responder in the aftermath of a traumatic situation). People who are highly empathic or who lack boundaries can easily be traumatized. Indirect exposure for highly sensitive people can create a serious trauma response because they lack the ability to create distance from the information.

Sometimes people are in drama therapy groups to treat trauma, and sometimes they are in drama therapy to work on other issues but have also experienced trauma. There are times when a participant has experienced trauma, but does not realize it because they have minimized the experience. It is also possible for a participant to experience trauma while they are in the course of drama therapy treatment. Whatever the origin or onset of the trauma, the therapist should be on the lookout for indicators, such as irritability, aggression, risky or destructive behavior, hypervigilance, heightened startle reactions, difficulty concentrating, isolation within the group, or a sudden, unexpected behavior change.

Environmental Triggers

Triggers are stimuli that remind the person of the traumatic experience. To help trauma survivors feel safe, the therapist needs to be aware of environmental factors that could be triggers. For example, a loud noise could trigger a startle response or a flashback. The sounds might be coming from outside or inside the drama therapy space: percussion instruments, balloons bursting, punch balls popping, cars backfiring, or something heavy being dropped. The sound might not even be loud; it could be a gentle sound effect tape of ocean surf. Another type of trigger could be certain smells, textures of materials or art supplies, or the sight of something associated with the traumatic experience. To avoid environmental triggers the therapist can bring out all the supplies within the space that might make a loud noise, have scents, have unusual textures, or are visually cuing like a play gun, knife, or costume. If someone finds something that might act as a trigger, that object can be put away and not incorporated into any sessions. While a therapist might be hesitant to ask about triggers, people who have had traumatic experiences are actually relieved to be asked and appreciate the opportunity to have some control in the therapy space.

Use of Touch

So many interventions in drama therapy include touch that drama therapists sometimes forget how much touch is involved. The NADTA code of ethics (2019a) requires therapists to get permission from participants before touching them or having them touch others. The code also mentions that there must be a therapeutic reason for the use of touch. This protects everyone from misunderstanding touch as a sexual come-on. Another reason to ask is to avoid triggering someone who has been through a traumatic experience. Even people who have experienced an upsetting situation that did not reach a level of trauma can be startled by an unexpected touch. When explaining an intervention, the drama therapist wants to identify where and how touch will be used. Following that, the therapist can ask if anyone would prefer not to be touched in this way. While doing interventions involving improvisation and physical play, in-the-moment check-ins about touch also avoid surprising participants.

Cognitive Concerns

Reading Ability

Assess the reading ability of participants before doing informed consent. Informed consent must be written at the reading comprehension level of the participant. If the participant cannot read, the therapist must read it aloud or provide it in a recorded format. When nonreaders are in a play and have lines to memorize, the script or parts of the script that the nonreaders are in can be recorded, or if the participant has a computer or iPad, they can use vocal software to play the script out loud.

Thinking Styles: Abstract Versus Concrete

Due to age, ability, medication, or diagnosis, some participants may have difficulty with abstract thinking. *Abstract thinking* is the ability to think about objects and ideas that are not physically present, use metaphors and analogies, substitute symbols for actual objects, persons, or meaning, and rotate objects in one's head without having it present. *Concrete thinking* is based in the body and the physical world. It is here-and-now thinking. All knowledge gained through the senses, experience, and experimentations are concrete.

Those who are new to drama often do better if they have costumes and props to use instead of imagining them. As they become more experienced, they start to be able to imagine costumes and props. Using concrete objects not only fleshes out the dramatic experience, it can be a bridge to abstract thinking. A concrete thinker acting out a meal might need to start using real food, then move to plastic play food, and finally create food through pantomime alone.

Drama therapy interventions involve concrete and abstract experiences. If participants in a group are a mixture of concrete and abstract thinkers, pairing concrete and abstract thinkers together in scenes can provide the concrete thinkers a model to help the transition from real to imaginary. Having a peer demonstrate an action through pantomime allows the concrete thinker to grasp the idea of using imagination more quickly. Because the essence of dramatic reality is moving from ordinary reality into dramatic reality, any kind of pretend work in dramatic reality helps develop abstract thinking ability. In a sense, drama therapy provides a continuum from concrete to abstract thinking that scaffolds thinking abilities.

Storytelling can be adapted to move along the concrete-to-abstract continuum. In the beginning, the storyteller can almost act out the characters of the story and use props and simple costumes to create images for the listeners. As time goes on, the storyteller can pull back to dialogue and description that is less physically active and more filled with metaphors and sensory images.

Participants can be involved in telling their own story, creating symbols, metaphors, and characters to represent the concrete. In *the six-part story method* (Lahad, 1992; Lahad, Shacham, & Ayalon, 2013), participants create a story by drawing pictures of six different aspects of the story: the main character, task facing the main character, things that hinder the main character, things that help the main character, the turning point of the main action of the story, and the aftermath or denouement. Fairy-tale components in the participants' culture bridge the gap between the concrete and the abstract. Originally, the method was designed to work with participants who have experienced trauma; making the connections between self and metaphor are not part of the treatment. However, if developing abstract thinking, the therapist can work with the participant to understand the connections between the characteristics of the participant and the characteristics created in the main character. As that character develops and becomes more fantastical, the character moves away from the concrete to become a projected abstract metaphor that can be used in therapy.

Similarly, theatre games like "the magic stick" or "the magic scarf" help with the transition from concrete to abstract thinking because there is an object in the participant's hand that can be seen in the space and used in place of the real object. The participant does not have to hold an image of the object in mind, it can actually be seen. This scaffolds the participant's ability to think metaphorically.

Working Memory

There will be participants who, due to brain injuries, substance abuse, or neurological disorders, have impairments in working memory that cannot be improved. These participants will need accommodations and adaptations in order to understand. Diagrams, pictures, and other visuals that keep information concretely in front of participants will help. Additionally, allowing participants to write information down, making it visual, can be helpful. Scripts developed from improvisations may be easier to memorize than ones that are given to the participant.

When an actor has great difficulty with memorization, a character can be created who reads from a notebook or clipboard as part of the action. For example, a police detective interrogating a suspect could have interview questions written in his notebook; an administrative assistant could have a clipboard to ostensibly make notes on that also has the actor's lines.

Sequencing

Damage to the frontal lobes or the cerebellum can cause difficulties with sequencing. Participants with learning disabilities, schizophrenia, Parkinson's disease, Huntington's disease, and working memory deficits also struggle with this. Sequencing can be supported through visuals and note-taking. As described in Chapter Three, directions can be given one by one, having the group complete each step before describing the next one. Drama games that build sequencing skills include "group storytelling," "fortunately/unfortunately," "Fedder's four," "hand-squeeze," "machines," "pattern ball passing," "people-shelter-storm," "scene using three props," "swoosh-bong," "spectrograms," and "zip-zap-zop."

Attention and Focus

Difficulties with attention and focus can be part of many diagnoses. Obviously, attention deficit hyperactivity disorder (ADHD) has these dysfunctions as major components. Depression, anxiety, schizophrenia, absence seizures, grief, bipolar disorder, learning disabilities, autism spectrum disorder, trauma and stress-related disorders, neurodevelopmental disorders, neurocognitive disorders like Parkinson's disease, Huntington's disease, Alzheimer's disease, and other types of dementia all involve attending and focusing difficulties. The drama therapist must understand whether it is possible to aid in the development of these skills or if one can only make adaptations without hope of change.

Again, visual aids can be helpful. They provide something to regain attention. There are theatre games where attention recall is an aspect of the game. Throwing a ball around a circle popcorn style requires attention to be focused and refocused as the ball goes from one person to the other. The "captain is coming" requires players to reattenuate to different commands. In "mirroring," players focus on a partner and must retain that focus. Other games like "who's the leader," "follow the leader," "yes-no-you," "1776," and "back-writing" can also develop attention and focus skills.

Lack of attention and focus can lead to safety concerns in a session. The drama therapist needs to be aware of the space and equipment in the room. If there is a tempting object like a bookshelf, toys on a toy-shelf, or recreational equipment in the room, those items might need to be covered up or removed. Prepare participants before moving into a new space, or they may be distracted by the novelty.

For example, a rehearsal room is very different from a stage. Check props or costumes that have parts like fringe, pins, zippers, or ties that could harm or distract participants. It can be helpful to make a checklist of distractors for certain participants that can be double-checked before they are scheduled for therapy.

Reality Testing

Reality testing is the ability to assess one's thoughts and emotions accurately and objectively, in order to be congruent with the outside world. Put simply, it is one's ability to see a situation for what it really is, as opposed to seeing it as what one hopes it would be or what one fears it is. It is also the ability to let go of assumptions that are incorrect in order to adjust one's thinking. This is different from everyday differences in perspective that one might have on social justice, economic, religious, or other cultural and personal issues. A deficit in reality testing is often associated with psychosis and personality disorders.

A participant whose reality testing is poor might have delusions of grandeur and believe in having powers or status that do not exist. Participants with poor reality testing may have fixed beliefs that they are unwilling or unable to reassess even in the face of contradictory evidence. Poor reality testing is more extreme than being in denial or being rigid. For example, a participant may believe he can psychically communicate with a movie star and that she psychically responds.

This type of participant may enter dramatic reality deeply and easily and not want to come out. Concrete closure can help bring them back to themselves, especially by following the scene immediately with a variety of deroling activities. In contrast, participants with poor reality testing may have difficulty entering and staying in dramatic reality. They cannot leave their own reality and go into someone else's or co-create another reality with a partner. They may need more distance. Storytelling, drama games, and movement-based bodywork can be more appropriate interventions for them than improvisational scenes. Seasoned drama therapists sometimes join in and play with delusions, but additional training is needed before an early career drama therapist tries this.

Drama games that could assist participants in developing better reality testing could be "two truths and a lie" or "to tell the truth." In addition, the group can practice going in and out of dramatic reality for short stretches of time in order to clearly delineate the boundaries for those who are fearful of losing themselves in dramatic reality and for those who have difficulty in leaving it. Discussions focused on the life-drama connection can help create distance and understanding. Deroling after each intervention and before leaving at the end of a session is of paramount importance, especially for participants whose boundaries between reality and fantasy are thin or porous.

Disorganized Thinking

Disorganized thinking falls along a continuum. At one end are people who have difficulty thinking in a clear, organized, and sequenced manner. They are in touch with reality and can tell a complete story that makes sense, but they tend to jump quickly from one thing to the next, not always in order. At the other end of the continuum are people whose thought processes are extremely disorganized and jumbled and not in touch with reality. Diagnoses tend to fall along the continuum depending on how the disorder impacts the individual's thought process.

Low			High
ADHD ASD	Depression Anxiety Stress	Severe Trauma Neurocognitive Disorders	Psychoses

Diagnoses like ADHD and autism spectrum disorders (ASD) are the least disorganized. When something interesting pops into their heads, they are easily distracted and follow that thought down a rabbit hole. The connections between the points of their story are there, but they are difficult to follow. This kind of thinking makes it difficult to solve problems or follow a process through from beginning to end.

People with diagnoses like depression, anxiety, and trauma have a different quality of disorganized thinking. Organized thought takes effort. It is a learned skill. When in a state of depression or anxiety, the mental energy to focus on organizing thought is not there. When telling a story, the storyteller's thoughts can be disconnected due to having to search laboriously for ideas, which just will not come. With more focus and energy, they can increase their organization and coherence of thought.

Severe trauma or neurocognitive disorders like Alzheimer's disease muddle a person's thinking. The disorganization is interconnected with their memory issues. Drama therapists do not always have the entire personal history of the client to put the pieces together and understand what the person is talking about. Because of the memory issues, skills that are gained can often be lost again.

At the other end of the continuum are thought disorders: psychotic conditions like schizophrenia, bipolar disorder, and dissociative disorder. In schizophrenia, for example, there is a lack of coherence of thought. It is very difficult for other people to understand how the thoughts are connected so what comes out sounds like nonsense or a word salad.

A number of the interventions that were mentioned for helping sequencing abilities would help with disorganized thinking by helping structure a clear narrative. Those interventions would include "group storytelling," "fortunately/unfortunately," "Fedder's four," "zip-zap-zop," and "yes-no-you." Systematic role creation could also assist in developing an organized method for thinking through a character, which could then be played out with instructions for the beginning, middle, and end.

Because people who have thought disorders have more complex struggles with thinking, simpler and shorter interventions are better. With less ability to sustain organizational thought, therapy must happen in shorter intervals. After participants are able to form coherent thoughts and language structures on a small scale, they can be challenged with interventions that are a bit longer and more complicated. However, because some of these diagnoses are so severe, patience on the part of the therapist is required. Movement forward can happen; it just will not happen quickly.

Language Comprehension

Children and people who have intellectual and developmental disabilities, language disorders, expressive and/or receptive communication disorders, and similar diagnoses often have language comprehension problems. These disorders are diagnosed in childhood, but can continue throughout adulthood. Many of these participants will not be coming to drama therapy to work on the language disorder, but on other issues, like social skills and emotional regulation. While it is important not to talk down to participants, it is possible to speak in simpler sentences with a less complex sentence structure.

Like second-language learners, participants, who have language disorders, need wait time so they can process the verbal and visual information they are receiving, decide how to respond, and express their response (receptive and expressive communication). Western cultures are always in a rush. They speak fast; they think fast; they jump into action. Most neurotypical people need between one and ten seconds to receive and respond to a question. If you sit in silence and look at the second hand of a clock for 10 seconds, it will seem like a long time! Participants with language comprehension problems need even more wait-time. Research (Duell, 1994; Rowe, 1986) found that if students were provided with more wait time after teacher questions and after student responses, the students actually began having real discussions and conversations. The class became more student-centered and less teacher-centered. Students started asking more questions of their own, proposing more experiments, and taking control of their learning. The same changes can happen in a drama therapy group when wait time is observed and adjusted to the needs of the participants.

Idioms are phrases that mean something different from the actual words in it. "Break a leg!" is a theatre idiom. It does not mean you are hoping someone breaks their leg. You are wishing them good luck. Participants who have ASD will have particular difficulty with idioms, because they tend to be concrete and specific in their understanding of words. People in the process of learning a second language have difficulties with idioms, too. While a drama therapist could include learning about and acting out idioms as part of a session, most of the time it makes sense not to use idioms in general conversation or instructions.

Other Adaptations and Accommodations to Consider

Developmentally Appropriate Interventions

Children

When choosing an intervention, the therapist needs to think about the cognitive level of development of the participant. Piaget, Vygotsky, and other developmental psychologists identified that different cognitive skills develop at different ages. However, individual children mature at different rates. Most 3-to-5-year-olds are capable of participating in dramatic play, but each will have different levels of attention span, social skills, and ability to handle complexity. If the therapist tries to introduce an activity that is developmentally too far above their skill levels, it may not be successful. Vygotsky (1978) always suggested that teachers aim to create a zone of proximal development. This means that the skill levels of the intervention should be just a little bit higher than the participants' current skills. In this way, participants do not get bored and are enticed to grow just enough to not become frustrated and fail (Bodrova, Germeroth, & Leong, 2013). The therapist also needs to think through the appropriate level of language to use (as mentioned in the earlier section).

In terms of physicality, young children's level of strength and coordination are still developing, so interventions need to be chosen to fit their physical abilities. For example, interventions that need upper body strength, balance, and patience like "trust falls" and "tangling" would be beyond their abilities. Games like "go," "bunny-bunny," or "chick-a-berry" that require split-second timing and multitasking are most likely not appropriate.

Older Adults

Assumptions are sometimes made that older adults do not have the physical capacity or the mental ability to engage in certain interventions. Older adults with normal cognitive and physical functioning are capable of doing any kind of drama therapy intervention that fits their treatment plan goals and objectives. Often older adults have experienced many losses of family and friends, of jobs and life roles. They need the socialization and connection that a drama therapy group can bring to make new connections and develop new roles.

There are physical challenges that can arise as one ages, such as neuropathy, arthritis, vision impairment, reduction in muscle mass, loss of hearing, loss of mobility, and lessening of the senses of touch, taste, and smell. Not every person experiences all of these challenges, but it is important for therapists to recognize when these challenges are impacting an individual's ability to participate. Simple adaptations can make a big difference. For example, participants with balance problems may appreciate sitting in a chair with arms. A wireless microphone can supplement the volume of voices, allowing everyone to hear what is being said.

The big obstacle when starting with older adults is convincing them to let go of their inhibitions and be silly, because they have had years of society telling them to act like adults. Outsiders who observe a drama therapy intervention may judge it as infantilizing; however, it is really up to the members of the group to decide whether or not they feel an activity is appropriate. There is a difference between being childlike and childish. Drama therapists should not be afraid to ask their older participants to enter the childlike space of dramatic reality, because this is where imagination, freedom, expression, and creativity are housed.

If adults have a neurocognitive disorder like Alzheimer's disease, they may struggle with certain interventions due to the memory issues and thought disorders involved in their diagnosis. The therapist can make many interventions work using appropriate adaptations. An important one is shortening the length of time of sessions. Adults with dementia have shorter attention spans and can easily become restless. Depending on the group, sessions may last anywhere from 15 to 45 minutes. The drama therapy group will most likely need to be kept small with four to six members, so less time is spent waiting for a turn. Concrete props and costume pieces will appeal to the senses and engage participants' interest. Visual aids are important as concrete reminders. Music is motivating and brings the group together, especially music that was popular at the time the adults were teenagers.

Animals

Animals can assist participants in a number of ways. Service animals are trained to work by providing tasks for individuals with physical, emotional and/or cognitive disabilities. Therapy animals are trained to provide support for participants within an educational, medical, or therapeutic environment. Animal assisted therapy utilizes animals as part of medical and psychological treatment. Emotional support animals (ESA) are not professionally trained and provide support by being physically present with the individual. ESAs require basic obedience training and are only for emotional or psychological support.

Service Animals

Service animals include dogs and miniature horses only. They are trained to perform tasks for individuals who use wheelchairs, who are blind or Deaf, who have medical conditions such as seizures, diabetes, and narcolepsy, and psychiatric conditions such as PTSD, OCD, and psychoses. It is illegal not to allow an individual into a therapy group because they have a service animal. It is also illegal to not allow the service animal into a session. Because service animals are protected by the Americans with Disabilities Act (ADA), handlers are not required to inform the therapist about them beforehand. One way to be sure you know about service dogs is to include a question about them in your intake or informed consent form. Legally, the therapist may ask only if the animal is a service animal due to a disability and what tasks the animal is trained to perform. For instance, the animal could be trained to alert the participant if a seizure is coming on. Due to ADA and the Health Insurance Portability and Accountability Act (HIPAA) requirements, the person does not have to tell you why the animal alerts nor does the animal need to demonstrate the task. The person can simply say, "It's task is to alert."

If another member of the group is afraid of or allergic to dogs or miniature horses, a clause in the ADA regarding reasonable accommodations says if there is undue hardship, or the handler is unable to regain control after the animal is disruptive, the therapist can request that the animal not be permitted in the space (EEOC, 2002). If someone can take an allergy pill and not be adversely affected, they are not considered facing an undue hardship. Notify group members about the service animal and request them to communicate as soon as possible if there is an undue hardship before the group meets so, if necessary, a discussion can be had with the handler before the day of the session. The other reason for notification is there may be more than one service animal in a group. In such cases, it is highly recommended that the therapist offers a time outside of the session for all the service animals and handlers to meet.

When one of the tasks of a service dog is to alert to biorhythm changes, you may want to check if another group member has similar symptoms as the handler, because the service dog may respond to similar changes in that group member. This does not happen often, but it can, especially in a setting where more than one individual is experiencing high blood pressure or anxiety-based symptoms. In addition, if the therapist knows there is a likelihood that an intervention could change the biorhythms of participants, it is important to let the handler know ahead of time, so that adjustments can be made for the service animal.

It may be important to notify a handler when the therapist is bringing in highly stimulating visual or auditory materials for the session. For example, the service animal may not have been around paint, brightly colored scarves, or drums. This allows the handler to decide if they want to come in early and introduce the materials to the service animal before the group begins.

Allow the handler to go over the rules of service animals for the group members at the first session. A well-informed therapist can do this if the handler is too anxious. Other group members need to know that while service animals are working, non-handlers are not allowed to touch, talk to, or make eye contact with the animal. To reduce the distraction of the animal, handlers are often willing to spend a few minutes with the service animal not working to allow others in the group to meet and greet the dog. The drama therapist also must remember that service animals are working while they are in session, and therefore not attempt to incorporate the animal into a drama therapy intervention. Because service dogs often are required to alert, you would not want them distracted by playing a part.

Therapy Animals

In contrast, therapy animals have no legal protection and are not required by law to be accommodated into a therapy session. Therapy animals belong to the therapist or volunteer, not to a participant. Training and registration programs are available for therapy animals, but the law does not require them. Recommended animals for therapy are dogs, cats, rabbits, rats, guinea pigs, miniature horses, miniature pigs, llamas, alpacas, and some birds. Therapy animals provide ego support and comfort. They are used in a variety of settings, including therapy offices, schools, libraries, retirement communities, nursing homes, and hospitals. In a drama therapy group, a therapy animal could be incorporated into a scene if it seems to be appropriate and not harmful to the animal.

Animal Assisted Therapy

AAT is always provided by a professional who has knowledge and training in the service area (physical therapy, mental health counseling, etc.), as well as training and knowledge about the specific animal being used. The work is always documented and evaluated. The therapist or the facility, in which the animal works, would own the animal. In AAT, the therapist uses the animal in goal-directed interventions with the participant. For instance, if an older adult needs to improve range of motion in their shoulder, an animal assisted therapist could have the dog fetch a ball that the older adult threw repeatedly during the session. It is more motivating to throw a ball for a dog than to do 20 sets of exercise repetitions by yourself. Drama therapists are more likely to use therapy animals than to do AAT.

Emotional Support Animals

ESAs only have legal rights to be in public housing and airplanes with documentation from a treating physician. ESAs can be any domesticated animal. ESAs are owned by the participant and not required to have any training. In order to qualify for an ESA a person must have a documented emotional disability (i.e., a DSM diagnosis). Drama therapists are not required to allow ESAs into therapy settings.

Conclusion

The job of the therapist is to serve the participants. One of the best ways to do that is to start where the participants are. If cultural humility, adaptations, and accommodations are not in the therapist's tool belt, meeting the participants where they are becomes very difficult. This chapter has focused on those tools. One of the core elements of cultural humility is the recognition of the ongoing process that requires working with open-mindedness. In no way can this chapter cover every adaptation or accommodation necessary for every culture or ability. A book could be written on each of the individual topics covered here. The hope is that the questions posed will be a springboard to launch you into your own explorations.

8

Ethics

The intent of this chapter is to address ethical issues related to treatment planning and intervention choices. It is not meant to be an in-depth exploration of all ethical issues in drama therapy; that would take an entire book. Many questions included in the drama therapy decision tree relate directly to questions of ethics or laws, reminding drama therapists of restrictions or parameters they might need to remember in relation to particular diagnoses or environments. For example, interventions involving touch might be counter to the rules and regulations of a prison or contraindicated for group members who have experienced sexual trauma.

This chapter will provide a brief overview of the differences between values, morals, ethics, and law to create a consistent use of terminology before going deeper into ethical and legal concerns that tend to come up for early career drama therapists. Although the chapter uses the North American Drama Therapy Association (NADTA, 2019a) code of ethics as a basis, the principles are consistent with most drama therapy organizations. As of this writing, the ethics around social media have not been specifically included in the NADTA code of ethical principles. In addition, institutions that drama therapists work in often have rules and regulations that also need to be taken into consideration when choosing interventions.

Cultural competency and diversity are often considered a part of ethics; sometimes they are dealt with as a separate entity. Because diversity covers such a wide field, those issues were given a chapter of their own (Chapter Seven). This chapter focuses primarily on the ethical principles that interact with drama therapy interventions.

The Difference Between Values, Morals, Ethics, and Law

When discussing ethics, the concepts of morals and values must be addressed. Although these three are often used interchangeably in nonprofessional discussions, they are not, however, the same. Values, morals, ethics, and laws at their most basic definitions are simply rules that individuals follow. The continuum runs from the individual (values) to the community (ethics). It is always important to ask if the dilemma being faced is housed in a value, moral, ethical code, or law, as the consequences for a violation can be significantly different. Important to note also is that sometimes a dilemma is not an ethical dilemma, but occurs because of poor clinical judgment on the part of the therapist.

Values

Values are the rules that we personally decide to follow. Values tend to be a personal judgment about the worth or importance of a matter or the way in which an undertaking should be done. Values can be in alignment with community morals or only in alignment with one's own beliefs. When one behaves in a way that is not congruent with one's own values, the consequence is usually feelings of guilt or disappointment in self.

Morals

Morals are the rules set by society and smaller personal communities, such as religious, neighborhood, and ethnic groups. Morals often motivate the creation of laws, but they do not have the power of legal consequences if they are broken. Members of a community tend to follow the group morals unless they are in rebellion against them. The consequence of behaving outside the boundaries of the morals of a community is often to be ostracized or shunned.

Ethics

Ethics are rules set by a professional community. The consequences of violating an ethical principle can range from censure to loss of credentials. There may be overlap between ethics, morals, and values; however, there may also be conflicts among the three. Frequently one is born into one's community and does not have a choice in terms of the morals that the community holds; however, one can choose one's profession.

Laws

Laws are set by city, county, state, and federal governments. They can be influenced by values, morals, and ethics in a democracy through voting for or against them. Individuals are required to follow the laws, regardless of whether or not they are in alignment with their personal values. Violating laws tend to have the most significant consequences, ranging from monetary fines to incarceration. For the purposes of the drama therapy decision tree, the primary focus in this chapter is on ethics.

Ethical Dilemmas

An *ethical dilemma* is a situation in which the therapist has to make a difficult choice that goes against an ethical principle. More often than not, ethical dilemmas pose a choice between multiple ethical principles or pit an ethical principle against a value, moral, or law. Because of that, resolving an ethical dilemma is not about making a decision that is right or wrong; it is about what Kidder (2009) terms a *right versus right* dilemma. Ethical dilemmas focus on the decision-making process and critical thinking. An ethical drama therapist thinks through each side of the dilemma to determine the best choice, considering the participants and all the variables involved. The resolution of an ethical dilemma is usually housed in good clinical judgement.

Every approach of drama therapy (e.g., developmental transformations, narradrama, psychodrama, etc.) inherently has ethical and/or legal issues that are built into it and must be thought through by the drama therapist. This does not mean that every drama therapy approach is inherently unethical. It means that any therapeutic approach has the potential for an ethical dilemma to surface because of the complexity of the techniques and the uniqueness of participants and their needs. Our recommendation is for drama therapists to examine each approach they use to proactively identify where ethical dilemmas may potentially arise.

Poor Clinical Judgment

Drama therapists can be practicing within ethical guidelines and still demonstrate poor clinical judgment. Suppose a drama therapist chose to play the drama game "bang!" with juvenile delinquents. In this game a player in the middle points to someone in the circle. The players on either side of the designee will turn and shoot at him with imaginary guns, and shout, "BANG!" If the designee does not duck fast enough and is shot, they are eliminated from the circle. This game warms up participants by getting them physically and mentally active, while promoting focus and attention; however, the game reinforces negative behaviors (e.g., violence and crime) that have landed them in trouble. Does using this intervention create an ethical dilemma? The ethical principles that would most likely relate to this choice of intervention would fall under the principles of responsibility or competence. If the drama therapist knows how to play the game correctly, has worked in the correctional facility previously, and has found no rules against playing that game, nothing about that choice is unethical. Playing the game might be unwise, in poor taste, or a matter of poor clinical judgment, but it is not prohibited. The hope of the authors is that through the use of the decision tree, drama therapists will think through their choices and make better clinical and ethical decisions.

Principle of Professional Responsibility and Respect

The principle of professional responsibility is the foundation for the entire code of ethics. The ethical elements most commonly associated with professional responsibility are *respect*, *honesty*, and *transparency* in order to safeguard participants from harm. Professional responsibility is related to patients' bills of rights, in that it focuses on working with participants in a way that is consistent with their legal rights and with respect for their unique personhood.

Another aspect of this principle is that therapists do not knowingly provide false or inaccurate information about themselves, their practice, and drama therapy. That includes explaining what drama therapy is and what participants will be doing, in language they can understand. The majority of participants are not going to know the jargon and conventions used in theatre and drama therapy. Terms like *blocking, distancing, crossing,* or *doubling* could be very confusing, even if used correctly in an explanation.

This principle is also about community policing. If a drama therapist sees another drama therapist practicing outside of any principle of the ethical code, the witness is encouraged to address the issue with the alleged violator, and if that does not work, the witness must report the incident to the NADTA ethics committee. Willingness to cooperate with ethical investigations on resolving violations either your own or that of others is an important aspect of being responsible.

In addition, professional responsibility is focused on the therapist understanding the institutional environment in which the work is being done and the cultural environment in which the participant lives. Without awareness of traditions, rules, and behavior codes within the various environments, the therapist can set up a situation in which a participant can fail, be humiliated, or become ostracized. One cannot respect and protect participants without an understanding of the social/political/physical world in which they live.

> **Choosing an Ethically Appropriate Intervention**
>
> *Principle of Professional Responsibility*
>
> - What is the interconnectedness between my choice of intervention and the rights of my participant(s)?
>   - o What are the ethical or legal standards that the approach or intervention choice could be at odds with?
>   - o What are the legal or civil rights of the participant and their limitations?
>   - o Is my choice of intervention cultural appropriation?

Interconnectedness Between Choice of Intervention and the Rights of Participant(s)

What Are the Ethical or Legal Standards That the Approach or Intervention Choice Could Be at Odds With?

There are aspects of interventions that can cross the line of ethical codes or laws, such as touch, the choice not to participate in an intervention, or use of recording devices. These are addressed in the decision tree under each section of the ethical principles. It is important to think about the interconnection of all the planned interventions and the participants in relation to ethics and laws.

What Are the Legal or Civil Rights of the Participants and Their Limitations?

By law, participants have basic rights regardless of where they seek treatment. Each institution will have its own patients' bill of rights. An institution can make its patients' rights more stringent than required by the law, but cannot make them less stringent, unless the law allows the institution to do so (e.g., prison, military, hospital). Drama therapists need to double-check the list of participants' rights where they work to make sure their choice of interventions is staying within those guidelines.

If working with a *mandated participant*, such as someone convicted of driving while intoxicated (DUI), a domestic violence perpetrator, or a participant sent to treatment by a court system, a drama therapist should check how long the participant will be required to attend therapy. Lack of awareness of participant time limits or release dates could create a problematic situation. For instance, the participant, the remaining group members, and therapist need to be prepared for appropriate termination. If a play is being rehearsed and the participant is released from required treatment before the performance, there could be a role left empty shortly before opening night.

If participants are in mandated treatment for domestic violence or sexual assault, there may be rules related to the kinds of behaviors allowed to be acted out. If the drama therapist is using an intervention like developmental transformations or psychodrama, the therapist will need to know what those banned behaviors are. The ethical dilemma for the therapist is the risk of setting up the participant for consequences from the legal system; however, not using an intervention or altering it might negate therapeutic benefits that could occur. Is it more ethical to break the institution's rules or the therapeutic contract?

Here is an example of an ethical dilemma of this kind: A drama therapist is working with an incarcerated population that is required to participate at all times in group by the formal rules of the institution or by the informal rules set up by the guards watching the group. There are times when inmates come to drama group sick or upset about something that happened prior to the group. If the inmate has poor emotional or behavioral regulation and is in a volatile mood, the inmate cannot leave, but should probably not participate until after calming down. An appropriate therapeutic response might be for the inmate to sit out until in a regulated state; however, obviously allowing someone not to participate could put that person at risk for punishment. One ethical change the therapist could make in the moment would be to choose an intervention involving actors and an audience. The upset participant could sit in the audience and watch. In doing this, participation is still happening, and the participant can partake in the discussion after the scene.

Rights can be involuntarily taken away, but they can also be voluntarily given up if one chooses to enter an institution that has specific rules and limitations on behavior. For instance, a religious institution might limit the types of content that can be explored or the language that can be used. A therapeutic community may have cardinal rules that cannot be broken, such as no violence, drugs, or sex. There might be prohibitions about acting out certain behaviors like doing drugs. The drama therapist must take all this into consideration when choosing or adapting an intervention.

Is My Choice of Intervention Cultural Appropriation?

There are differing opinions about whether tools and techniques from one culture should ever be used by a therapist from another. If drama therapists are going to use therapeutic arts from another culture, it must be done for a valid reason and with respect for the culture of origin. The choice of the cultural tool must be consciously made to address specific therapeutic needs. For example, using a folktale from a culture to which group members belong could be more appropriate than using an unfamiliar folktale. However, the therapist must understand all the cultural implications of the tale's symbolism and cultural referents so as not to create confusion.

From a different perspective, a specific culture may have a problem with the use of an intervention because it contradicts their beliefs. If therapists are not of that culture, they may not be aware that the intervention is inappropriate. For instance, some religious denominations do not agree with the use of folktales or legends that involve magic, wizards, witches, or pantheons of gods. Acting out stories about Harry Potter, Hercules, Odin, or Gilgamesh would not be acceptable to them; neither would creating a story in the style or structure of a legend or myth. Even yoga might be considered inappropriate by religious groups who view it as a Hindu ritual. In such instances, the drama therapist would want to avoid physical warm-up activities that incorporated yogic postures or pranayama (breathing).

Drama therapists need to have appropriate training to be competent with the tool or technique being considered and understand its history and cultural meanings. Respect can be shown by making sure an educational component is incorporated to make sure that participants not of the culture of the tool or technique understand why this technique is being used, along with its origins and purpose within its original culture. A tool from another culture must not be changed or Westernized to fit purposes they were not intended for or to make the therapist look "cool" and "with it."

Responsibility and Social Media

As of this writing, social media is not addressed in the NADTA ethical code, however, it does relate to the principle of responsibility. A therapist cannot post anything on social media that is untruthful about a participant, another drama therapist, or drama therapy itself. Memes can be problematic, because they tend to make satirical or overgeneralized claims. Sharing opinions about participants, colleagues, or drama therapy approaches also falls into the category of "untruthful," because opinions could be taken as facts.

Principle of Competence

The principle of competence relates to professionals' abilities to do their jobs with proper skills and awareness, staying within their appropriate scope of practice, experience, and education. Competence does not mean expertise; it refers to the foundational level of ability to do a proper job. Competence includes three subcategories: *competency of knowledge and skills, cultural competency*, and *professional development*. Cultural competency was addressed in Chapter Seven.

Competency of knowledge and skills includes knowing the theories and skills involved in improvisation, drama therapy approaches, theatre techniques and therapeutic processes. Of crucial importance are the skills of group facilitation, which are developed through the internship process. The abilities to listen, engage in discussion and debate, and highlight insight without bias can guide participants to make discoveries for themselves.

Developing competency is an ongoing process. Professional development is an attitude of being open to learning from every situation one is in and from every person with whom one works. Ongoing training (continuing education) needs to be done to continue to keep skills sharp and to add to one's knowledge base, particularly in regard to new discoveries, theories, and techniques.

Principle of Competence

- What do I do if I choose the wrong intervention?
- What if I am working with a new population?
- What if a theatrical performance is appropriate for the participants, but I have never taken a directing class?
- What if a devised performance is appropriate, but I have never taken a playwriting class?
- How much training should I have before I use specific interventions?
- Am I aware of the most current information about a diagnosis, theory, treatment, or intervention?

What Do I Do if I Choose the Wrong Intervention?

The first thing to do if you make a mistake is to take responsibility for the mistake. Mistakes happen, and they are not unethical as long as you openly take responsibility with other members of the treatment team and the participants. There is nothing wrong with saying, "I'm really sorry. I made a mistake." It will not destroy people's trust in you; in fact, honesty and transparency often increases their trust in you.

The second thing to do is to go back and look at your decision-making process to see where you erred. If you notice the mistake in the middle of the intervention, it is acceptable to stop the intervention. Explain to the participants that they are not doing something wrong, that you have mis-chosen the intervention or given the wrong directions. Then either clarify the instructions, or switch to a different intervention that better addresses the issue.

If you are not sure why an intervention is not working, consider the following:

- Is the distancing of the intervention off in relation to the psychological distance of the participants in the moment?
- Has enough trust and group cohesion been built between the group members and between the group members and the therapist to do this intervention?
- Have the participants been warmed-up enough to do this task?
- Is there an environmental factor that has not been taken into account?
  - Someone is missing from the group, and the group dynamic has shifted.
  - The weather is affecting group members or the therapist.
  - There are bad smells or noise pollution in the space.
  - National or international news has upset group members.
  - A loss (death, firing, quitting) has happened to group members.
- Do participants first need to learn a skill, in order to scaffold a skill needed for this intervention?
- Is the intervention too complex for an aspect of their:
  - Executive functioning
  - Emotional regulation
  - Behavioral regulation.

What If I Am Working With a New Population?

If you are starting a job with a population you have never worked with before, this can compromise your competence. You need to find a supervisor who has experience with this population to be a guide and sounding board before and while you are beginning with this new group. You also need to read about the needs of this population in general. First-person narratives of people who have this diagnosis can help a great deal because they are speaking about the symptoms, feelings, and experience from their own perspective. Books about drama therapy and other creative arts therapies about this population may have great ideas to pull from. Librarians can be very helpful if you are not sure where to turn to for resources. If your library does not have the books you want, most libraries have interlibrary loans. There is a bibliography of drama therapy books, journal articles, and chapters on the NADTA website at https://www.nadta.org/what-is-drama-therapy/Resources.html, which is periodically updated.

What if a Theatrical Performance Is Appropriate for the Participants, but I Have Never Taken a Directing Class or Directed a Show?

Directing is an important theatre skill. It involves many demanding tasks, including appropriately analyzing and understanding the script, coaching actors, blocking and creating effective stage pictures. When a therapeutic performance is publicly produced, other theatre artists, such as costume, set, and lighting designers, might join the production team. Directors need to communicate effectively with stage managers, designers, theatre technicians, and promoters. If you have not had any directing training, it would be important to either take a basic directing class or ask a local director who has a good reputation if you could be assistant director for a show or two.

What if a Devised Performance Is Appropriate, but I Have Never Taken a Playwriting Class?

Devising a play is writing a play with input from actors, usually improvisational input, which is then scripted. It is important for a drama therapist who is working on a devised or ethnographic play to understand play structure. While many theatre students do not take playwriting at the undergraduate level, often they take courses in dramatic structure, script analysis, or dramatic literature. Some writers interested in autobiographical or self-revelatory plays have said that memoir, autobiography, or self-in-narrative classes have helped them shape their plays. These types of courses can be helpful. However, the authors recommend the study of playwriting as a skill-set on its own as a play has its own specific dramatic structures and requirements. If such courses are not available, books like *Ethnotheatre: From Page to Stage* (Saldana, 2016), *Naked Playwriting: The Art, the Craft, and the Life Laid Bare* (Downs & Wright, 2004) or *The Writer's Journey: Mythic Structure for Writers* (Voegler & Montez, 2007) can be very helpful. The commonality of these books is their clarity on how to structure a performable piece of drama.

How Much Training Should You Have Before You Use Specific Approaches?

In terms of postgraduate training, there is a gold standard and an acceptable standard. The gold standard involves using an approach under direct supervision of an expert therapist. The supervisor can correct the natural beginner's mistakes and offer guidance. Sometimes this happens during an internship or in a work environment. In terms of psychodrama, developmental transformations, and other approaches, it can also happen within ongoing long-term training groups. There are certifications or credentials available for approaches like psychodrama, playback theatre, developmental transformations, or rehearsals for growth, which are earned after completion of a certain number of workshops/trainings, assignments or tests.

The acceptable standard would involve going to a daylong workshop or weekend intensive to learn the basics of a technique. This does not provide real-life hands-on experience with participants, but with appropriate ongoing supervision, this kind of training can be enough to learn a technique. Another acceptable option would be to read about a technique and have conversations with individuals who use it regularly. When beginning to use it with participants, do so under appropriate ongoing supervision. Please note, this paragraph has not been about learning and trying out complex approaches, but about singular techniques. Complex approaches really need to be learned through the gold standard approach.

Am I Aware of the Most Current Information About a Diagnosis, Theory, Treatment, or Intervention?

Continuing education begins the day after a student graduates. Information about diagnoses, theories, treatments, and interventions are changing constantly. New interventions are being created that make old ones outdated. For example, in substance abuse treatment for several decades there was a theory about the family roles played in an addict's family. The roles were the scapegoat, the clown, the rebel, the hero, the mascot, the rescuer, the doormat, the adjuster, the bully, the last hope, and the lost child (Wegscheider, 1981). For most of the 1980s, 1990s, and early 2000s this family role theory was the guiding principle for working with adult children of alcoholics (ACoAs). However, subsequent research (Vernig, 2011) has not substantiated that these roles are valid or that ACoAs play these roles. This means that if a drama therapist working with ACoAs uses these roles in therapy, there might be little therapeutic benefit.

Alternatives to interventions can be created that work as well or better than older standard interventions. An example of this is trauma treatment. For years the only effective method of dealing with trauma was to have the trauma survivor tell the story of the trauma over and over until the trauma became habituated and lost its power over the person (Hermann, 1992). This process is painful, and because of that many participants do not finish treatment. However, there are now other treatments like Eye Movement Desensitization and Reprocessing (EMDR) (Marich & Danzinger, 2017; Shapiro & Forrest, 2004), yoga and neurofeedback (van der Kolk, 2014), drama therapy (Sajnani & Johnson, 2014), dance/movement therapy (Chaiklin & Wengrower, 2015), and art therapy (King, 2016) that have provided alternatives. Therapists who do not complete continuing education will not learn these new and improved ways to help their participants. In addition, when a drama therapist is licensed, continuing education becomes a legal requirement to maintain licensure.

Principle of Confidentiality

Similar to continuing education, confidentiality is both an ethic and a law. For drama therapists, it is about more than the protected health information collected on participants. It is about the security we use to store and share information about creative works. It relates to the creative processes that are developed in group. It is also about how we properly inform participants about the lack of confidentiality in public performances. It is important to note, informed consent will be referred to in this section, however, a more detailed discussion of informed consent will follow. Confidentiality cannot be discussed without first noting the federal regulations in the United States under the Health Insurance Portability and Accountability Act (HIPAA), the Family Education Rights and Privacy Act (FERPA), and Title IX.

Principle of Confidentiality

- What are the legal aspects of confidentiality?
    - HIPAA
    - FERPA
    - Title IX.
- What confidential information could a participant potentially share within an intervention?
    - Check-ins
    - Projective interventions
    - Improvisational scenes
    - Nonfiction interventions
    - Devised, ethnodrama, or autobiographical therapeutic performance
    - Discussions after interventions about the life-drama connection.
- What are the potential dilemmas between confidentiality and
    - Public Performance
    - Filmmaking/Recording/Photography
    - Public Displays of Creative Work
    - Projective Interventions
    - Storage of Participant Artifacts.
- Social Media
    - Have you addressed participants about taking cell-phone pictures or recording self or others in group or in rehearsal/performance?
    - Have you addressed participants about posting to social media?

Confidentiality Laws

HIPAA

The Health Insurance Portability and Accountability Act of 1996 is meant to protect health insurance coverage and personal health information in terms of its integrity, confidentiality, and availability. This means that before information is shared between institutions, doctors, therapists, and so on, a written permission form must be signed by the participant. What is important for drama therapists to know is that anything created artistically, because it is related to a therapeutic need, is considered protected health information (PHI). Photography, filming, public performance, drawings, anything created by individuals or the entire group is bound by the rules of confidentiality and privacy. This means in order to perform a play; written permission must be obtained. A participant's choice to perform is not enough to imply consent to release PHI (see Principle of Informed Consent below).

Storing Creative Work

HIPAA has rules for how to secure participant records. With written documentation, security is easily provided by multiple passwords and encryption. With creative work, particularly that which is three-dimensional and not digital, following the security rules can be more difficult. The easiest way to deal with this is to take a picture of the work and have participants take the work home with them. This option would be contraindicated if the creative work should not be seen by someone who lives with the participant or someone who may come into their living space.

Typically, participant records are accessible to anyone on the treatment team; however, creative work can be misinterpreted by those who lack the training or experience to interpret it. Records must be maintained, depending on the state, from five to ten years. HIPAA requires six years of record maintenance. At the end of that time, records are usually destroyed. Destroying a written participant record and destroying participant creative work is a very different experience. Therefore, what will happen to the creative work and the records ultimately should be included in the informed consent.

FERPA

The Family Education Rights and Privacy Act of 1974 protects the privacy of students' education records. This covers grades and academic work, as well as aspects of student life, such as mental health referrals, behavioral infractions, and financial aid. For students who are under 18, their parents hold the rights to their educational records; after 18 or once enrolled in higher education (regardless of age) the rights belong to the students themselves. Knowledge of FERPA is important for drama therapists working within a school system outside of the counseling center. Information revealed in an anti-bullying workshop in an elementary school to anyone, other than the children in the workshop or the parents of the children, without written permission, would be a violation of federal law. Information could be given to the principal, counselor, or teacher (who were not in the room at the time) only on a need-to-know basis; if it is not need-to-know information, it can be given out only with written permission of the parents of that student.

Need-to-know means the information is essential and necessary. The information must be facts only, not interpretations of facts. An example of need-to-know information would be if a male student disclosed that he was being bullied during an anti-bullying workshop. That information could and should be shared with the school counselor. If it is disclosed that a student who sits next to this boy in a class has been bullying him, the drama therapist could tell the classroom teacher to no longer have these students sitting next to each other. However, under need-to-know, the reason why they should no longer sit next to each other should not be disclosed. Need-to-know is separate and different from duty-to-warn requirements.

Title IX

Title IX of the Education Amendments of 1972 (2018) states: No person in the United States shall, on the basis of sex, be excluded from participation in, be denied the benefits of, or be subjected to discrimination under any education program or activity receiving federal financial assistance (para. 2). The most common Title IX issues that therapists deal with are sexual harassment, sexual violence, and gender-based discrimination, rather than aspects of the act like sports funding and discrimination. Only faculty, staff, and students at a university in the United States are mandated reporters for information they hear about a possible Title IX violation.[1] This means a therapist does not need to share any identifiable information to the Title IX office outside of the type of incident that occurred. If a drama therapist is not working in the counseling center but teaching experiential methods, and a student discloses a violation during a class exercise, regardless of licensure or certification, the drama therapist is a mandated reporter. The drama therapist is only a confidential reporter if working for the counseling center of the university.

Confidentiality in Drama Therapy

Confidentiality must be kept by the therapist. When working with groups, therapists should explain the importance of confidentiality to the group members and request that they also keep group information confidential; that is, what is disclosed in group should not be repeated outside of group. However, the therapist should also add that confidentiality cannot be guaranteed, since confidentiality could be breached by anyone in the group.

In traditional group therapy in which participants are talking about their issues directly, it is obvious when they are sharing about themselves. However, in drama therapy, participants sometimes share information without realizing they are sharing, because in addition to direct talk and discussion, improvisation and other projective techniques are used. This is why it is so important to address this in your informed consent.

The first time personal information will be shared is during check-ins. Typically, participants are asked to report on how they feel at the moment or what their experience has been between sessions. When a check-in is play-based, as opposed to round-robin report, a participant may initially make the choice not to share an incident. However, playing lowers a participant's defenses and can allow the participant to slip into sharing before really being ready. This type of response to play should be addressed in informed consent prior to the start of the group so the participant is aware of this potential. What is problematic is not the slipping into sharing. The problem occurs only when the participant does not realize there is a possibility that this might happen.

Interventions on the nonfiction side of the drama therapy pie are more likely going to expose personal information, but personal information can also be shared unconsciously through fictional interventions like improvisation and other projective techniques. There is nothing wrong with this, as long as the participant realizes in the moment that this is happening. However, there are instances when a participant might not want to share something like HIV status or might not be emotionally ready yet to share information like having been raped. By the time the group gets to improvising a scene or creating a sandtray, participants may have forgotten the information about self-disclosure that was in the informed consent form. It then becomes incumbent upon the drama therapist to remind them about this before beginning the intervention, so any disclosure will more likely be done willingly and knowingly.

Personal disclosure is definitely involved in the creation of a devised play, ethnodrama, or autobiographical therapeutic performances (ATP) done as part of drama therapy. In the process of devising a play, personal stories are often shared and improvised. Remind participants that they are the playwrights and if they want something they shared to remain confidential, they can delete it from the script, or it can be fictionalized so it is untraceable back to them.

Ethnodrama is created from interviews. Ethnodramatists need to evaluate their transcripts to be sure they are accurate and allow the interviewee an opportunity to clarify any aspect of what was said or request that certain information not be included. While ethnodramas are typically nonfictional in nature, interviewees could request that aspects of their story be fictionalized, or their names changed to protect their anonymity. ATPs are developed through a therapeutic process. Both the process and the end product need to be communicated to participants, who are going to be brave enough to share their healing process with others. Whichever type of performance is being created, participants need to know how much they will be expected to reveal to other group members and ultimately to an audience.

Confidentiality, Drama Therapy, and Public Performance

When participants give consent to be involved in a public performance, they must be made aware of two considerations that impact the limits of confidentiality. The first is that even though the participants may understand they are sharing information with the audience, they need to know that the audience is not bound by confidentiality. Audience members could share any information that they receive during the performance with other people. For instance, a coworker of a recovering addict could be invited to a performance about addiction and recovery. The coworker might share the information with the participant's boss the next day. This could be problematic with the participant's continued employment, or it could result in the boss making a comment in the break room in front of a number of other coworkers that reveals the participant's status to everyone on the job. In this case, confidentiality has not been broken, because once information is made public through the public performance, confidentiality is no longer protected under the law or ethics.

The other consideration regarding public performance is making sure the participants understand that the audience may not react the way they expect. Participants may feel incredibly empowered to share their coming out or HIV status while creating the play with a supportive group and therapist, but nothing guarantees that audience members will not laugh at the wrong places. They could also react with horror or anger at the actors and the information being disclosed in the play. What had been an experience of empowerment during rehearsals can become an experience of rejection and pain in performance.

Many participants in therapeutic theatre performances are new to the theatre and do not know what to expect. As long as they are aware of the worst-case possibilities and acknowledge that they have been warned by signing the informed consent form, the therapist can prepare for all eventualities. In the vast majority of cases, the worst-case scenario will not happen, but if it does, the participants will not be taken by surprise.

Confidentiality and Filmmaking/Recording/Photography

Filmmaking and photography are similar to performance in that the creative work becomes public; however, there is less control over who sees the work. A live stage performance can be limited to friends, family, and specific individuals who are invited, but with performance in the digital era, films and photos can be sent far and wide. This is true whether the original work is filmed and posted on YouTube or is a recording made for archival purposes.

Another possible dilemma is that film, recordings, and photography can be altered. This could be experienced as a devastating betrayal, if a participant was visiting YouTube or another form of social media and saw a mockery made of a performance or personal disclosure. This kind of alteration cannot be controlled once media is posted publicly; therefore, the therapist needs to make participants aware of digital manipulation as a potential risk in terms of informed consent.

Confidentiality and Public Displays of Creative Work

When artwork is displayed, confidentiality is broken when participants sign their work with their own names and/or have an identification of their personal information on a plate beside the work. A more confidential option could be displaying work anonymously or under a pseudonym. Thought should also be given by the therapist about which piece of work is chosen for display. It is possible that there is verbal or visual participant information in the work that could break confidentiality. There could also be the projection of emotional material displayed in the work that the participant might not want to disclose. This occurred in an art show at a school where one of the authors worked. Students created family portraits in art class. One student's drawing revealed that she lived in a single parent home. She had not disclosed this to any of the other students. When they saw it, they ridiculed her.

There is also the possibility that images in artwork could be incorrectly interpreted. A drawing made by a participant in a therapy group, who is feeling overloaded by responsibilities, could symbolize the situation by drawing multiple representations of themself going in different directions. This could be misinterpreted as a diagnosis of dissociative identity disorder.

Similar to recordings being altered, displayed creative work can be damaged by mistake during transportation or while being put up or taken down. If the gallery space is not carefully watched, the work could be vandalized or destroyed. This can be a heartbreaking experience for the artist and could feel like a personal violation.

Confidentiality and Projective Techniques

As all drama therapists know, there is no way to predict what kind of confidential information will be shared when using a projective technique. Therefore, participants need to be made aware of the limitations of confidentiality in terms of revealing unconscious information. While drawing, dancing, or improvising, the participant may share something unconsciously through the projective technique that they do not realize they are disclosing. When others see what the participant has made, they may recognize its meaning. There is also the possibility that they project their own problems onto the work and misunderstand its meaning. In the case of participants who are still early in treatment or who have not yet disclosed a great deal of information to the group, the drama therapist might want to remind participants to only share what they feel comfortable disclosing to the group.

Information of an intention to do harm to self or others might appear in a projective technique. The therapist would then be required to break confidentiality and report to an appropriate authority. In addition to information about projective techniques in the informed consent form, therapists may want to remind participants about the duty to warn before doing projective techniques by specifically listing items that by law are mandated to be reported.

Confidentiality and Safety of Participant Artifacts

The biggest thing to think about is when an intervention results in the creation of an artifact that the therapist does not have room to store and that is not safe to be stored in the participant's residence. For instance, a huge three-dimensional object could reveal unflattering opinions about the participant's parents or siblings that would be seen if taken home. Even though the therapist has carefully made the decision for the intervention based on the clinical needs of the participant, the intervention becomes a poor choice if there is no safe place to store the artifact. Something that cannot be stored may have to be destroyed. Destroying a therapeutic artifact potentially could be contraindicated for the mental health of the participant. If the participant were part of destroying the artifact with the therapist, it would need to be done in a therapeutic manner. This type of ethical dilemma needs to be thought through ahead of time.

If stories and discussions are recorded for a devised play or an ethnodrama, the therapist needs to think about how the material will be transcribed. If the therapist is not going to do the transcription and is going to hand it to a transcribing professional or a volunteer, then participants must be made aware of this in their informed consent. The transcriber must be made aware of the confidential nature of the material and agree to keep confidentiality through a signed agreement. Once the material is transcribed, the tapes should be destroyed or completely erased. Materials should not be placed on Google Docs or YouTube for editing, sharing, or transcription purposes, as these platforms are not secure enough and, therefore, not HIPAA compliant.

Confidentiality and Social Media

As of this writing, there are no specific NADTA ethical codes around social media use; however, a lot of confidentiality can be broken by the use of social media. Uploading photos or videos of participants to any kind of social media platform (Facebook, Snapchat, Twitter, Instagram, etc.) breaks confidentiality, unless you have written consent. This includes any work done in sessions or rehearsals, cast parties after performances, or any other occasion. This consent must be given before the photo or video is taken, not after. While this may seem old fashioned to digital natives, it goes straight to the heart of the principle of confidentiality because social media goes out to thousands of people, and once it is posted, it cannot be totally retracted. Just deleting a post does not mean it is gone; it still remains somewhere up in the cloud forever.

One of the risks of confidentiality is letting participants bring cell phones or other recording equipment into your therapeutic space. Everyone's confidentiality could be broken if photos or videos are taken and uploaded to social media. If the therapist knowingly allowed the recording devices into the therapy space, and the facility is under HIPAA jurisdiction, the therapist, rather than the participants, would be held accountable for the lapse in confidentiality.

If the therapist knowingly shares a post that breaks confidentiality, the therapist can be held to the same standard as the person who posted the material originally. If the person who posted is not a member of NADTA, they will not be filed against for an ethical violation because they have not officially violated confidentiality. A drama therapist, however, still can be held accountable because they are supposed to know better.

Principle of Informed Consent

Informed consent at its most basic is how therapists let participants or their guardians know exactly what is going to be taking place during the therapeutic process. This can include techniques and interventions to be used, the benefits and risks of engaging in the therapeutic process, and specific to creative arts and drama therapy, a description of performance, use of projection, and how that relates to confidentiality, as well as the issues with photography, recording, and other media. All these are interventions that are not typically used in traditional psychotherapy. More typical content for informed consent, like fee schedules, cancellation policies, and storage of records, should also be in this document. In addition, participants need to know they have the right to refuse to join in any activity or comply with any request made of them in therapy.

Informed consent must state any limitations to confidentiality, such as harm to self or others, and child or elder abuse. Whenever informed consent is being used in an institution, such as a prison, court order for mental health, or a system such as the military, information must be included about the limitations of confidentiality that those entities have mandated.

The therapist must specify whether assessment or therapy is being done. This is because there are different aspects of confidentiality between situations of assessment and therapy. Insurance companies and other appropriate entities will need to have access to information from assessments. If this is not mentioned, then a separate release must be created and signed to give permission for release of information when it is sent to those entities. If research is being done as part of clinical practice, participants must be made aware of this in the informed consent form, along with specifics about the research and who to contact if they have a question or complaint.

All of this must be written in accessible language for the participant. For instance, if the participant is a child, use simple sentences and words that they can understand. If the participant speaks a different language, have a copy of the form translated into that language as well as providing one in English. If the participant has an intellectual or developmental disability (IDD), break down the information into accessible language on that specific person's reading and cognitive levels. If the participant cannot read, the form must be read to them.

Participants need to remember what they have agreed to, so a copy of the informed consent form, signed by them and the therapist (and their guardian, if necessary), should be given to them. The therapist keeps a signed copy as well. When working with individuals who require guardians' consent, the guardian also needs to have a copy of the informed consent form.

If by chance the direction of therapy changes midway through treatment and different types of interventions will be used, an updated informed consent form will need to be signed. For instance, if there was no plan to do a public performance and suddenly the whole group decides that they want to devise a play, the original consent form would not have listed the benefits and risks of performance or the limits to confidentiality of public performance. Informed consent addendums are not the same as retroactive consent. They must be signed prior to the change being made.

Therapeutic Interventions Used as an Assessment

Therapeutic interventions often provide assessment-type information to a therapist (see Chapter Six and the six-key model). It is important for drama therapists to be transparent about how assessment-type information gathered through the intervention will be used. All good therapists gather information throughout the therapeutic process. This information helps them know when participants have achieved treatment goals or objectives and when a new therapeutic objective needs to be addressed. This gathering of information is different from formal assessment. In traditional therapy, assessment and therapeutic interventions look very different. Since the difference may not be obvious in drama therapy, participants must have clarity when one or the other is being done. For example, role method can be used as an intervention or an assessment. The way role method is done in a session as an assessment or as an intervention can appear identical to a participant, even though the purposes are different. All ethics codes state that participants must be aware of which way an intervention is being used.

A drama therapist may be doing an assessment, and the participant has a therapeutic response to it. While the drama therapist as assessor has a responsibility to make sure the participant is safe, they should not fall into the role of therapist at this time. The informed consent is what allows the drama therapist to keep these roles separate.

Cell-Phone Pictures or Recordings

Most therapists recognize the importance of gaining informed consent when they are recording or photographing participants; however, in this day and age of ubiquitous cell phones, most people make an everyday practice of photographing themselves, their friends, their pets, and their food. Participants involved in drama therapy sessions, rehearsal, or performance may pull out their cell phones to take a picture or record something they feel is interesting or memorable without giving it a further thought. It will be necessary to mention in informed consent that taking photos or recordings of self and others during the group is not permitted because of confidentiality. It may also be necessary to ask participants to leave their cell phones at the door in a basket or box at the beginning of a session. If a therapist becomes aware that a participant has filmed or taken a photograph, it is the therapist's responsibility to delete it. Even if the participants involved in the photo/recording say it is OK, the deletion must still happen because consent cannot be given after the fact, only before.

Informed Consent Checklist

- Name of client/participant
- Name of therapist and credentials
- Contact information
- If a drama therapist is not yet an RDT, they need to include the name, credential, and contact information of their supervisor.
- Number of sessions per week/length of session
- Cost per session
- Cancellation policy
- Medical issues the therapist should be aware of and how to help
    - o Emergency contact for a family member
    - o Emergency contact of the doctor or specialist.
- Storage of records
- Description of drama therapy in general
- Types of interventions expected to be used
    - o Benefits and risks of those interventions
    - o Use of touch.
- Use of projective techniques
- Photography/videotaping
- Right of participant to refuse
- Limitations of confidentiality
    - o Harm to self
    - o Harm to others (duty to warn)
    - o Child or elder abuse
    - o Institutional, system, or insurance limitations
    - o Performance and recordings.
- Doing assessments
    - o Who will the assessments be shared with?
- Doing research
    - o What are you studying and why?
    - o Who to contact if you have questions.
- Requirements regarding HIPAA, FERPA, Title IX, as relevant

Principle of Physical Contact, Role-play, and Other Drama Therapy Activities

This principle covers the maintaining of good professional boundaries with regard to the participants' best interests and safety. Many therapeutic codes of ethics forbid or seriously limit the use of physical touch for good reason. The therapist is in a position of power in the therapist-participant relationship, and in the past, there were therapists who abused that position. In drama therapy touch is involved in a number of interventions and can also happen unintentionally. Participants in drama therapy always have the right not to be touched if they do not want to be. A statement to this effect needs to be in the informed consent form, so participants are aware they have this choice. The drama therapist is responsible for knowing how touch or the lack of touch is going to change an intervention. If the drama therapist knows that an intervention has the potential to lose some of its therapeutic value due to lack of touch requested by the participant, other techniques that would be better suited may need to be used. For example, "tangling" is a wonderful metaphorical intervention to allow participants to experience that all life's tangles can be untangled if they are worked on long enough. Participants also experience that often one is not able to see all sides of an issue and needs to have help from others who have a wider or different perspective. Someone who has been sexually abused or who is claustrophobic might feel extremely uncomfortable in a tangle. Those concepts can be experienced through different interventions.

Principle of Physical Contact, Role-play, and Other Drama Therapy Activities

- What do I do when my place of employment dictates the rules of physical contact or other aspects that could come up from drama therapy interventions?
- What do I do when a participant does not disclose issues around physical contact until already involved in an intervention?
- What is the relationship between my own personal beliefs about physical contact and my choice of interventions?
- What do I do when a participant appears to be manipulating physical contact with other participants or with the therapist?
- What do I do if a participant does not have the emotional or behavioral regulation to refrain from inappropriate touch?

Rules From Place of Employment

There are regulations against touch, language, or specific behaviors in certain environments. The boards of education in certain school districts have mandated that no student may be touched. Many therapeutic communities have similar rules. This can be frustrating if, for instance, the therapist's value is that participants need to be touched or need to be allowed to express themselves without censorship. If there is a rule prohibiting touch or certain types of self-expression, the therapist must abide by it. A conversation with a supervisor or director about the therapeutic benefits of the banned behavior could explore whether an exception could be made with the general rule. For instance, if physical contact is forbidden, permission could be made for high-fives to be given for a job well-done.

Late Participant Disclosure Regarding Physical Contact Issues

Sometimes participants do not realize what their reaction will be to an intervention until they are in the middle of it. For instance, participants who are claustrophobic might believe they can "tough it out" making a plaster of Paris mask. Their motivation might be that everyone in the group is going to have one, and they want one, too. However, when the materials are put over the participant's face, mouth or eyes, they could become panicky. This could be due to a general feeling of helplessness or a flashback to a time when they were held captive in a closet as a child. Whatever the reason, the therapist must stop the intervention for that pair and make sure the panicking participant is safe.

There could be a situation in which participants who do not like each other are paired together. They may refuse to work with each other or begin to work together, then start acting out or making excuses. Depending on the maturity and cognitive capabilities of the participants, the therapist can help them work together by monitoring them closely, offering suggestions for adapting the activity so that there is no touch, or by making another accommodation. If the partner conflict looks like it is going to create a big blow up, taking the path of least resistance and switching partners might be easier. It is not appropriate to deal with an individual behavior issue in front of the whole group. Intervening later with the acting-out participant will avoid reinforcing the behavior with negative attention from the group. A therapist not only has to pick which battles to fight, but also to think about how to use them from a therapeutic perspective to benefit all the participants.

Therapist's Personal Beliefs Involving Touch

Often therapists' personal beliefs about the appropriateness or inappropriateness of touch influence their choice of interventions. For example, an inexperienced therapist who feels touch in therapy is inappropriate may avoid improvisational interventions, such as developmental transformations, contact improvisation, or a game like "elbow-to-elbow." Decisions about interventions need to be based more on the participants' needs than on the tentativeness of the therapist.

On the opposite end of the spectrum, there are therapists who strongly believe in the healing power of touch; however, touch might be contraindicated for certain participants with a history of trauma or a particular diagnosis. An obvious example of this would be participants with autism spectrum disorder (ASD) who are tactilely defensive. Any kind of warm-up with touching, tagging or other kinds of physical contact might not be the best way to engage them. For a less obvious example, methadone and heroin addicts often have a residual sensory sensitivity to touch. Sometimes during use and often during withdrawal, participants will feel as if their skin is crawling with insects. Certain kinds of touch used in an intervention, even after they are clean and in recovery, can restart the crawling sensation. Adderall can have a similar effect, especially for individuals who are taking it simply as a stimulant, as opposed to as a doctor-prescribed medication for attention deficit hyperactivity disorder (ADHD). Any time an intervention involving the potential of physical contact is chosen, the therapist must evaluate if touch is clinically in the participants' best interests.

Touch can help create a safe environment, facilitate an emotional bond, and increase the feeling of trust between therapist and participant leading to deeper self-disclosure (Pattison, 1973; Raniszewska-Wyrwa, 2014). It also has been shown to reduce anxiety and muscle tension as well as increase well-being (Carneiro et al., 2017). Comfort with the use of touch in therapy varies from culture to culture. Understanding whether your participants will feel positively or negatively toward touch is an important part of cultural competence. Participants from cultures that are generally comfortable with touch may feel comfortable with interventions that use touch.

On the negative side, touch can intensify an existing trauma and can be misinterpreted. Touch has been a controversial topic not just in drama therapy, but in all forms of psychotherapy. The authors are not taking a stand on whether or not touch is ethical. Our stand is that anytime touch is introduced into the therapy session, drama therapists need to ask themselves what the purpose and therapeutic benefit of the touch is. Making sure that the choice is driven by the needs of the participant rather than driven by personal feelings allows a drama therapist to ethically use the healing power of touch.

Participant Manipulating Physical Contact

There are participants, particularly people with Down syndrome and Williams syndrome, who because of their IDD, are prone to hug everyone. This section is not about these participants. There are other participants who have difficulty with healthy boundaries who will manipulate for attention and touch other participants and the therapist. Their attention-seeking rarely makes them favorites within a group, as other group members often feel overwhelmed, invaded, and sometimes attacked by them. Their behavior probably originally developed from a very functional desire to get their attention needs met, but perhaps because those needs were ignored, they now overly seek physical connection.

The therapist must set boundaries with the manipulative participant in terms of physical touch and also must make sure that others in the group are not put at risk. Therapists want to be careful which interventions they choose in order to help set up boundaries. Interventions can be adapted to make them safer. One intervention that might help set up personal space within a group is the game "find the space." Group members move around the room at different speeds determined by the leader and find spaces where other people are not. This requires taking stock of where you are, where the other people are, where they are moving, and where you are moving. After the game, the therapist has that intervention to refer to in terms of keeping group members in their own spaces during other activities. If this intervention is not concrete enough, the therapist could try "hula hoop/bubble walk" to create clarity on what amount of area denotes personal space around each person.

"Pop toob conversation" is an intervention that helps develop an understanding of personal space. Invented to teach college students about consent, it can be used to explore any type of boundary issue. Group members pair up and each one gets two pop toobs (plastic accordion fidgets). The group decides on a scenario and a specific distance between the actors in which that conversation will be enacted. Each pair acts out their scene using the pop toobs to demonstrate the distance they are from each other. Then the scene is replayed: once with the pop toobs shortened and once with them extended. The group discusses the three versions of the scenes; often in the discussion group members realize that the shorter the distance, the more uncomfortable they felt, and the longer the distance, the safer they felt. When the participant with the boundary problems does a scene, the leader would make sure that pair acted out a scene that needed more space.

Participants Without the Emotional or Behavioral Regulation to Refrain From Inappropriate Touch

As mentioned at the beginning of the last section, there are participants who because of a cognitive or emotional disability have difficulty understanding boundaries and therefore have difficulty refraining from inappropriately touching other participants and the therapist. These participants need to learn about social boundaries for their own protection. People who walk around the streets hugging other people can be arrested for sexual harassment. They could also hug the wrong person and end up kidnapped or assaulted. For these participants, any of the games just mentioned followed by group discussion would work to teach boundaries and understand appropriate social interactions with acquaintances and strangers.

Conclusion

Ethics is the last chapter of this book, not because it is an add-on, but because it overarches all decisions a therapist makes. Not every principle in the NADTA code of ethics was explored because the focus here was on ethics and the appropriate choice of intervention. The principle of teaching and training has been observed throughout the writing of this book. We have tried to ensure that we were providing the most foundational, accurate, objective, and current information. When current research was not available, as in our search for information about executive functioning, we did our best to synthesize what was known.

The principles of professional relationships and research were also not specifically addressed in this chapter. A number of aspects of professional relationships were covered in Chapters Seven and Eight. In Chapter Seven the diversity aspects of professional relationships were addressed. Other parts of those principles seemed to be outside of the scope of this book.

This book's purpose is to provide a systematic way to approach drama therapy practice in order to integrate the knowledge that drama therapy students have learned in their education and training. Drama therapy is presented to students through courses, conferences, workshops, and books. Sometimes a variety of approaches are taught separately and without reference to the phases of the psychotherapeutic process, as if any technique or intervention can be used at any time for any problem. The reality is Emunah's five phase model of drama therapy (2020) is the only model that is in alignment with the developmental approach of the psychotherapeutic process (Yalom & Leszcz, 2005).

As mentioned in the prologue, when different sets of information are taught at separate times, they are not always integrated for the student in a later class.

The use of the drama therapy pie in conjunction with diagnosis, phase, and psychological/aesthetic distance allows drama therapists to practice competently and integrate their knowledge of drama therapy and psychology into the therapeutic process. The use of the drama therapy decision tree helps drama therapists generalize their therapeutic understanding, so they can create integrative treatment plans, apply drama therapy interventions systemically, and evaluate the therapeutic work that has been done.

NOTE

1. At the time of publication, new regulations for Title IX were implemented, no longer requiring faculty, staff and students to be mandated reporters. However, the new regulations are being challenged in the US court system.

Appendix A
The Drama Therapy Decision Tree

DIAGNOSIS

What Symptoms Are the Participant Experiencing?

- What are the specific criteria of the DSM?
  - Which of the specific criteria does the participant meet?
- What are the observable and/or self-reported dysfunctions?
- Are there global treatment symptoms to address (i.e., executive function, locus of control, etc.)?

What Are Driving the Symptoms?

- Are there physical causes?
- Are there social or economic causes?
- Are the symptoms being reinforced?
- Is the participant on medication for this diagnosis?
- Is the participant on medication for other medical or mental health issues?
- Is there drug/alcohol/caffeine/tobacco use? Contraindications?

Do the Symptoms Allow the Participant to Avoid or Gain Something?

- If the symptoms allow the participant to avoid something, what is it?
- If the symptoms allow the participant to gain something, what is it?
- Can drama therapy address the underlying issue?

What Cultural Aspects Need to Be Considered With the Diagnosis?

- Cultural aspects and traditions of the participant that need to be considered:
  - Ethnicity/Nationality
  - Religious Affiliation or Spiritual Affinity
  - Gender Identity
  - Gender Expression
  - Sexual Orientation
  - Socioeconomic Status
  - Educational Attainment
  - Work-related Identity
  - Political Affiliations or Beliefs
  - Geographical Culture
  - Language.
    - Native/Secondary Language
    - Dialect
    - Localisms.
  - Intersectionality of any of the above
- Are there symptoms the dominant culture sees as abnormal, but the participant's culture sees as appropriate behavior?
- Are there behaviors that are being identified as symptoms that really are a representation of being misunderstood or discriminated against by authorities in the dominant culture?
- Are there symptoms outside of the standard diagnostic criteria that are only associated with or normally expressed in the participant's culture related to this diagnosis that also need to be addressed or acknowledged?

Questions to Identify Initial Goals for Treatment Plan

- Priority: What are the potential harmful consequences that could occur if a particular symptom is not addressed first?
- What symptoms need to be dealt with in order to create an impact on the participant's day-to-day living or to jump-start success/improvement?
- Are there any symptoms that need to be addressed before other symptoms can be addressed (learning skills, scaffolding understanding, or accepting given life situations, etc.)?

- Are there goals that can address multiple symptoms?
- Are there symptoms that need to be addressed now, but must be addressed by a different professional?

Is Drama Therapy Appropriate to Address the Treatment Goals?

- What is the rationale for why/how drama therapy would be useful for these goals and objectives?
- Is there research that supports using drama therapy for this diagnosis?
- Does the drama therapist have experience using drama therapy with this diagnosis? If not, where is there information? Who could supervise/consult?
- If this is group therapy, do participants in the group have more than one diagnosis?
  - o If this will cause a problem, how can that best be dealt with?

PHASE

What Phase of Treatment Is the Participant in?

- Has the participant been in drama therapy before?
- What emotional and behavioral signs does the participant exhibit?
  - o Which phase do these emotional and behavioral signs fit into?
  - o Are there treatment goals that need to be addressed for the participant specific to the phase?
- If doing group treatment, is the group starting now, or is it an ongoing/open group?
  - o If the participant is joining an open group, are other participants in multiple phases? If so, how do you plan to deal with that?
- What issues addressed in this phase are part of normal group development that do not need to be specifically addressed in the participant's treatment goals (i.e., developing a therapeutic relationship, developing trust between group members, understanding group rules, etc.)? These issues will need to be taken into consideration when choosing an intervention.

Important Questions to Keep in Mind During the Course of a Phase

- What are typical signs that participant/group is ready/not ready to move to the next phase?
- What are signs that participant/group has regressed to a previous phase?
  - Does therapist know why this has happened?
  - Does this regression impact treatment goals or intervention choices?
- Using the above information, identify the phase the participant/group is in.

Outside Influences Affecting Treatment Outcome

- Are there any outside influences impacting participant in personal/work life?
- Potential group dynamic issues:
  - Open versus closed group
  - Attractions between participants
  - Animosities between participants

The Interaction of Diagnosis and Phase of Treatment

- How does the current diagnosis present in this phase of treatment?
  - What interventions might be useful for this diagnosis in this phase?
- How does the current diagnosis present differently in different phases of treatment?
  - What interventions that might typically be done in the current phase, need to be saved for a later phase, or not done at all?
  - What interventions would be contraindicated in certain phases?
- Are there issues in the diagnosis that could cause difficulty in a specific phase (i.e., dependent personality disorder causing difficulty in termination phase?)
- What issues involved in the diagnosis might impact the length of the phases?

PSYCHOLOGICAL DISTANCE

Participant's Overarching Predisposition for Psychological Distance

- Is the participant typically intellectual and unemotional most of the time?
- Is the participant typically highly reactive and emotional most of the time?
- Is the participant relatively balanced between emotion and thought most of the time?

Emotional Regulation Abilities of the Participant and Group

- If participant/group is typically under- or overdistanced, does this need to be added as a treatment goal?
  - o If yes, what is the urgency? Does a treatment goal need to be added immediately to the treatment plan, or can it wait until other goals have been addressed?
- What is the participant's/group's psychological distance upon arrival at the group today?
- Is something different about the participant's/group's emotional regulation today?
  - o If so, what is different?
  - o What is the reason?
    - ▪ Do they know?
    - ▪ Do you know?
- Are you able to adjust the participant's/group's distance through the warm-up? If not, how can you address this distancing challenge?

The Interaction of Diagnosis, Phase, and Psychological Distance

- Is participant/group under- or overdistanced because of:
  - o Medication
  - o Diagnosis
  - o Usual psychological distance.
- Is the psychological distance related to the current phase?
  - o Just beginning

- Transitioning between phases
- Nearing termination
- Terminating.

THE DRAMA THERAPY PIE

Choosing an Appropriate Intervention

Fiction or Nonfiction Interventions

- Is the participant/group better able to work with fiction (acting through metaphor/distance) than nonfiction (acting out their own lives)?
- Does the participant/group have enough reality testing to remain psychologically intact if working on traumatic or highly emotional material about their lives?
- Is there enough trust and respect in the group to work with nonfiction material in terms of the vulnerability that comes with personal disclosure?
- What kind of setting are you in?
  - In a prison, jail, or detention center, what are the contraindications of nonfiction work?
    - Disclosure by participant of crime that must be reported?
    - Participant disclosing information to an "enemy" inside or outside the group (inmate or staff) that could be used against them?
    - Other?
  - In an educational setting, a drama therapist's contract is often focused on psychoeducational goals rather than therapeutic ones and often class periods are between 45 and 60 minutes. Fictional work tends to provide more containment so students can transition quickly from group to academic class. What is your situation?
  - In long-term residential settings (i.e., treatment centers, nursing homes, etc.) trust may have already been established among residents, and facility staff could provide safe containment to process issues between therapeutic groups. Nonfictional work benefits from the continuity provided by long-term groups. What is your situation like?

Process-Oriented or Presentational Interventions

- Is the group open or closed? If the group is open, it will be very difficult to create, rehearse, and perform a play since members of the group will change.
- Would the participant/group be able to handle presenting a play in front of an audience?
- Do participants have the social skills to work with each other in rehearsals?
  - o If social skills need to be worked on, would rehearsals provide enough practice in working with others?
- Do participants have the emotional regulation to deal with nerves and stage fright?
  - o Is sharing the participant's/group's story part of the healing that needs to happen?
  - o Have the participants processed the emotional material to be included in the play enough so that they would not be overwhelmed by a new discovery about themselves during the performance?
  - o Are there diagnoses in the group where having a wider audience (if doing a play) would be contraindicated, for instance, for participants who are histrionic or attention-seeking?
  - o Do the participants have enough ego-strength to deal with the rehearsal and performance process?
  - o If autobiographical, does the material being presented in a play have aesthetically pleasing aspects that would be accessible to an audience?
    - ▪ Autobiographical or solo performance requires more ego-strength than a fictional or group performance.
    - ▪ All plays inherently have a level of fiction and distance, depending on the use of metaphor to express emotional truths. The use of metaphor supports participants who have less ego-strength.
  - o Is there a space in which you can perform?
- Are there ethical concerns in having participants perform?
  - o Are there HIPAA concerns or permissions needed regarding participants performing for each other or a larger audience?
  - o Are there issues of confidentiality, such as parental or guardian permission in order to perform?
  - o Are participants survivors of domestic abuse who need their location kept secret from their abusers?
- Does the aesthetic distance inherent in the type of performance intervention fit with the group needs?
- Would the participant/group do better with process-oriented work?

  - o Do you have enough time to spend in self-discovery and play development (if it is a devised play), or would you need to jump right into mounting a production?
  - o Do you have participants who would not want to perform in a play?
    - ▪ Too young
    - ▪ Not confident enough
    - ▪ Not enough emotional regulation
- Are the issues that need to be worked through severe? If so, staying focused on process might be more useful.
- Life-drama connection (i.e., talking about the intervention afterwards):
  - o Can the participant/group readily understand the life-drama connection, or does it need to be made concrete for them?
  - o Do you want to focus the discussion on the process of the drama therapy work, the outcome of the drama therapy work, or both?

What Kind of Embodiment Do the Participants Need?

- Self:
  - o Does the participant need hands-on practice/rehearsal to incorporate skills?
  - o Does the participant need to be embodied in order to understand or gain insight?
  - o Does the participant need to learn give-and-take with other group members?
- Others:
  - o Will watching others' enactments provide enough distance for the participant to understand what is going on?
  - o Will watching others' enactments provide opportunities for the participant to learn through the observation process?
- Objects (props, costumes, masks, drawings, etc.):
  - o Are objects needed in order to engage participants in therapy?
  - o Are objects needed to ensure metaphor (distance) for participants?
  - o Are objects needed to ensure understanding (concreteness) for participants?
  - o Are objects needed to ensure focus/attention of participants?

The Interaction of Diagnosis, Phase, Psychological Distance, and the Drama Therapy Pie

- Interventions:
  - o What interventions are effective in the current phase of treatment?

  - o Given those interventions, which are appropriate considering the diagnosis of the participant?
  - o Are there specific distance needs?
- Do you want the intervention's aesthetic distance to match or balance the participant's current psychological distance?
  - o What type of embodiment does the participant need?
  - o Should these interventions be fictional or nonfictional?
  - o Can this be addressed through the warm-up or will more of the session need to be adjusted to create balance?
  - o How much of the life-drama connection needs to be addressed in discussions about the intervention during closure?
- What additional issues relating to diagnosis can be addressed in different phases as treatment progresses for the participant?
  - o Can nonfictional interventions be used?
  - o Does metaphor provide a wider/more complete view through which participants can see and address their dilemmas?
- Can the level of discussion about interventions become more abstract, less distanced, or more personal as participants develop insight, or due to diagnosis does discussion need to remain concrete and distanced?

Global Outcomes With Drama Therapy

Creativity

- Is there anything within the diagnosis that hinders creativity?
  - o If so, do you want to include a creativity treatment goal?
- Does your participant/group believe that they are creative?
- Does your participant/group feel afraid/unconfident in a specific art area?

Spontaneity

- How much spontaneity does your intervention require?
  - o Is there anything within the diagnosis that hinders spontaneity? If so, do you need to:
    - ▪ Include a spontaneity treatment goal?
    - ▪ Include teaching of spontaneity skills?

Sensory Integration

- If your participant has sensory integration issues, what do you need to consider in regard to:
  - o Intervention materials?
  - o Interventions themselves?
  - o Included as part of the treatment plan?

Metacognition

- Is your participant/group capable of metacognition? Populations such as people with IDD, dementia, and young children may have difficulty talking about the life-drama connection.
- Does your participant/group overintellectualize? Do they become easily overdistanced?
  - o If so, they may sound like they understand the life-drama connection and the emotions discussed, but in reality, they do not. You may want to consider emotional explorations versus metacognitive ones after interventions are over.

Emotional and Behavioral Regulation

- If the participant/group are not able to regulate emotions and behaviors, could interventions trigger them to:
  - o Lose emotional control?
  - o Lose behavioral control?
  - o Dissociate?
- If the participant/group are overregulated in terms of emotions and/or behaviors, could interventions trigger them to:
  - o Shut down emotionally?
  - o Refuse to participate?
- Does a treatment goal need to be added to help improve regulation?

Locus of Control (LOC)

- Does your intervention require a more internal or external LOC?
- Does your participant/group have a more internal or external LOC?

- Are there group dynamics that come into play if the LOC is widely different between group members, leading to a lack of understanding of each other's points of view?
  - o A group could have a similar LOC due to past experiences or diagnoses.
  - o A group could have a mix of LOCs.
  - o One group member could be extremely internal or external in their LOC in comparison with the rest of the group.
- Do you want to incorporate changing your participant's/group's LOC as part of the treatment plan?

Check-ins

- Will your check-in work best if it is ritualized and the same each session, or will it work best if it is varied each time?
- Does your check-in need to be direct, or can it be metaphorical?
  - o Can your group understand metaphor?
    - ▪ If not, can they learn to use metaphor?
- Does your check-in need to be embodied?
  - o Can embodiment wait for warm-up?

Warm-ups

- How much warm-up is needed?
- Does your intervention later in the session need a specific warm-up?
- Is the warm-up the intervention?
- What do you need to consider regarding diagnosis and individual factors?

Closure for Interventions

- What type of closure is appropriate:
  - o Verbal Processing
  - o Action
    - ▪ Ritual.

- Have the participants who were involved in the intervention been deroled?
- Have the participants who were witnesses to the intervention been deroled?
- How much metacognition is needed in order to wrap up?

Closure for a Group Session

- When does the session end? Is there enough time left to do the wrap up that was planned, or does it need to be changed?
- What type of closure is appropriate:
  - o Verbal Processing
  - o Action
    - ■ Ritual.
- Have the participants who were involved in the intervention been deroled?
- Have the participants who were witnesses to the intervention been deroled?
- How much metacognition is needed in order to wrap up?

Six Keys to Assessment

The First Key: Passage—Entering and Exiting Dramatic Reality

- Can the participant enter dramatic reality easily?
  - o If not, how difficult is entering? Is it possible at all?
  - o What could be the obstacle?
- Can the participant exit dramatic reality easily?
  - o If not, how difficult is leaving?
  - o What could be the obstacle?

The Second Key: The Quality or Style of Dramatic Reality

- Can the participant remain in the dramatic reality for the whole enactment?
  - o If not, what could be causing the difficulty of staying engaged?

The Third Key: Roles and Characters

- What roles does the participant tend to play?
  - o Is the participant's role repertoire wide or narrow?
    - ■ If it is narrow, do the roles all relate to one theme?

- Can the participant develop three-dimensional characters?
  - If the participant is stuck in only creating archetypical roles, what is the block to fleshing out those roles into characters?

The Fourth Key: Content Patterns: Plot, Themes, and Conflict

- Does the participant have an ability to enact a wide variety of content and conflicts?
  - If not, is the limitation due to lack of life experience?
  - If not, is the limitation due to fear of conflict?
  - If not, is the limitation due to fear of expressing certain emotions that might come up?
- Is there a common theme to the types of plot/conflicts the participant enacts?
  - If so, what issue(s) could be expressed by this theme?

The Fifth Key: Response to Dramatic Reality From the Outside

- Is the participant able to witness other group members?
  - If not, why?
- Is the participant able to distance self from the characters and themes enacted?
  - If not, why?
- Is the participant able to discuss what has gone on in scenes?
  - If not, why?
- Is the participant able to hear and accept the audience response to their performance and/or discussion comments?
  - If not, why?

The Sixth Key: Meta-Reality or the Unmanifested Subtext

- Is there any subtext or meta-reality in this scene?
  - If so, what is it? Can you verbalize it, or is it still just a feeling?

Questions to Ask Yourself About Cultural Competence

- What are my culture biases and assumptions?
- Am I aware of how the privilege/power I hold impacts the therapeutic relationship?
- What assumptions am I making regarding the culture of my participant based on prior experience with a similar culture or a similar participant?
- What aspects of my participant's cultural background is most central or important to them?
- In concrete terms, what have I done to get to know the participant and better understand their perspective?
- Do I have any strong positive or negative feelings toward my participant?
    - How are those feelings impacting the therapeutic relationship?
- Am I aware of my participant's perceptions of me?
    - If so, what are they? If not, I need to ask.
    - How are those perceptions impacting the therapeutic relationship?
- Am I aware of all the intersectionality this participant has?
- In concrete terms, what am I doing to show respect for my participant?
- What am I doing that does not show respect for my participant?
- What are the cultural components of the drama therapy intervention?
    - Is there a conflict between the intervention and the participant?
    - Is there a conflict between the intervention and the participant's culture?
- Does the participant's culture make the participant vulnerable to specific dangers?
    - Prejudice from other community members or a hate group?
    - Deportation?
    - Other governmental or legal ramifications?
        - Will a certain intervention heighten those dangers?

Checklist to Ask Yourself About Cultural Appropriation

- Is my practice or artifact from the dominant culture?
    - If not, to which ethnic/racial/cultural group does the practice or artifact belong?
- Is the group that the practice or artifact belongs to oppressed?
    - If yes, does my use of the practice or artifact continue the oppression?
        - Does the practice or artifact represent the oppression?
        - Does the practice or artifact represent defiance of the oppression?
- Apart from any clinical benefit to my participants, how do I benefit as the therapist from using this practice or artifact?

- o By making money from selling it?
- o By being seen as "cool" or "with it"?
- o By being seen as "cutting edge"?
- Why might my use of this practice or artifact make someone from the ethnic, racial or cultural group of origin uncomfortable?
- How did I learn about this practice, tradition, or material?
  - o Did I find this on the internet?
  - o Did I read about it in a book?
  - o Did I learn this in a training or class?
    - If I did, was it assessed by the presenter for cultural appropriation?
  - o Did you learn this from practitioners from the culture of origin?
    - Did they give me permission to use it?
    - Were there any restrictions or guidelines?
- How am I honoring and giving credit to the group that created this practice or artifact?
- Am I modifying the practice or artifact?
  - o How am I modifying it?
  - o Why am I modifying it?
  - o What legitimizes my changing it?
  - o Am I explaining this to my participants?

Adaptations and Accommodations

Cultural Adaptations and Accommodations

- What is the native language of the participant?
  - o If it is not the dominant language the group is being conducted in, how well does the participant comprehend that language?
  - o Does the participant need a translator?
  - o Could the language barrier be addressed through:
    - Simpler words?
    - More use of gestures?
    - Intervention adaptation or accommodation?
- Is there a change that would make the intervention more culturally relevant?
- If cultural appropriation could be an issue with a participant or participant group, what can be done to change it?

Diagnosis/ability Adaptations and Accommodations

- Is the participant functionally mobile?
  - If there is a mobility impairment, what assistance is needed?
    - Gross motor functioning
    - Ability to walk
    - Ability to sit and stand
    - Ability to make large arm or leg movements
    - Coordination/balance
    - Fine motor functioning
    - Gripping/holding
    - Writing/painting
    - Use of tools or machinery
  - Does the participant use a mobility device? If so, what adaptation is needed for interventions?
  - Does the mobility device itself impose limitations?
  - Does the mobility device create safety issues?
- Does the participant have a vision impairment?
- Is the participant deaf of hard of hearing?
- Does the participant have a medical diagnosis that could impact the group or session?
- Are any participants survivors of trauma?
- Are there cognitive adaptations that need to be made to interventions because of the diagnosis or an identified disability?
  - Can the participant read?
  - Is the participant able to think abstractly, or are visual and/or concrete materials necessary to clarify instructions?
  - Does the participant have normal working memory?
  - Can the participant keep sequences in order?
  - Can the participant focus/attend, or is the participant easily distracted?
  - What is the participant's reality testing?
  - Does your participant have organized or disorganized thinking processes?
  - What is the language comprehension of the participant? Will you need to use:
    - Simpler sentences?
    - Simpler words?
    - Avoid idioms?

Other Adaptations and Accommodations

- Is the intervention age/ability appropriate?
- Is there a service animal that needs to be incorporated into therapy?

- o Service animal
- o Therapy animal
- o Animal assisted therapy
- o Emotional support animal.

Accommodations and Adaptations Checklist for Participants With Hearing Loss

- **Communication and Instruction Accommodations**
  - o Obtain participants attention before speaking
  - o Frequently check for understanding
  - o Repeat and rephrase information
  - o Enhance speech/lip reading conditions (keep hands away from mouth, no gum, etc.)
  - o Clearly enunciate and allow extra time for processing information
  - o Use visual aids
  - o Present information in a simple, structured and sequential manner
  - o Provide handouts with basic information/outline for the session.
- **Physical Environment Accommodations**
  - o Reduce auditory and visual distractions (carpet, sound dampening materials, reduced sound of AC units, etc.)
  - o Bright lights
  - o Room set-up to allow for everyone to be facing each other
  - o Visual alarm systems.
- **Intervention Adaptations**
  - o Break up instructions, step by step
  - o Give many breaks during session (listening with a cochlear implant, lipreading, etc. is exhausting)
  - o Provide supplemental materials
  - o Have a partner/buddy system
  - o Add other sensory components to a traditionally verbal intervention.

Adapted from Johnson, Benson and Seaton (1997) *The IEP Checklist*

Choosing an Ethically Appropriate Intervention

Principle of Professional Responsibility

- What is the interconnectedness between my choice of intervention and the rights of my participants?
  - o What are the ethical or legal standards that the approach or intervention choice could be at odds with?
  - o What are the legal or civil rights of the participant and their limitations?
  - o Is my choice of intervention cultural appropriation?

Principle of Competence

- What do I do if I choose the wrong intervention?
- What if I am working with a new population?
- What if a theatrical performance is appropriate for the participants, but I have never taken a directing class?
- What if a devised performance is appropriate, but I have never taken a playwriting class?
- How much training should I have before I use specific interventions?
- Am I aware of the most current information about a diagnosis, theory, treatment, or intervention?

If Your Intervention Is Not Working Consider the Following

- Is the distancing of the intervention off in relation to the psychological distance of the participants in the moment?
- Has enough trust and group cohesion been built between the group members and between the group members and the therapist to do this intervention?
- Have the participants been warmed up enough to do this task?
- Is there an environmental factor that has not been taken into account?
  - o Someone is missing from the group, and the group dynamic has shifted.
  - o The weather is affecting the group members or therapist.
  - o There are bad smells or noise pollution in the space.
  - o National or international news has upset group members.
  - o A loss (death, firing, quitting) has happened to group members.

- Do participants first need to learn a skill, in order to scaffold a skill needed for this intervention?
- Is the intervention too complex for an aspect of their:
  - o Executive functioning?
  - o Emotional regulation?
  - o Behavioral regulation?

Principle of Confidentiality

- What are the legal aspects of confidentiality in terms of:
  - o HIPAA
  - o FERPA
  - o Title IX.
- What confidential information could a participant potentially share within an intervention through:
  - o Check-Ins
  - o Projective Interventions
  - o Improvisational Scenes
  - o Nonfiction Interventions
  - o Devised, Ethnodrama, or Autobiographical Therapeutic Performances
  - o Discussions after interventions about the life-drama connection.
- What are the potential dilemmas between confidentiality and
  - o Public Performance
  - o Filmmaking/Videotaping/Photography
  - o Public Displays of Creative Work
  - o Projective Interventions
  - o Storage of Participant Artifacts.
- Social Media
  - o Have you addressed participants about taking cell-phone pictures or recording self or others in group or during rehearsal/performances?
  - o Have you addressed participants about posting on social media?

Informed Consent Checklist

- Name of client/participant
- Name of therapist and credentials

- Contact information
- If a drama therapist is not yet an RDT, they need to include the name, credential, and contact information of their supervisor.
- Number of sessions per week/length of session
- Cost per session
- Cancellation policy
- Medical issues the therapist should be aware of and how to help
    - o Emergency contact for a family member
    - o Emergency contact of the doctor or specialist.
- Storage of records
- Description of drama therapy in general
- Types of interventions expected to be used
    - o Benefits and risks of those interventions
    - o Use of projective techniques
    - o Use of touch.
- Photography/videotaping
- Right of participant to refuse
- Limitations of confidentiality
    - o Harm to self
    - o Harm to others (duty to warn)
    - o Child or elder abuse
    - o Institutional, system, or insurance limitations
    - o Performance and recordings.
- Doing assessments
    - o Who will the assessments be shared with?
- Doing research
    - o What are you studying and why?
    - o Who to contact if you have questions
- Requirements regarding HIPAA, FERPA, Title IX, as relevant.

Principle of Physical Contact, Role-play, and Other Drama Therapy Activities

- What do I do when my place of employment dictates the rules of physical contact or other aspects that could come up from drama therapy interventions?
- What do I do when a participant does not disclose issues around physical contact until already involved in an intervention?

- What is the relationship between my own personal beliefs about physical contact and my choice of interventions?
- What do I do when a participant appears to be manipulating physical contact with other participants or with the therapist?
- What do I do if a participant does not have the emotional or behavioral regulation to refrain from inappropriate touch?

Appendix B
Global Outcomes Connected to Drama Therapy Intervention Suggestions

To help connect drama therapy interventions with the global treatment outcomes (behavioral regulation, cognitive regulation, emotional regulation, locus of control, physiological regulation, and social-emotional reciprocity), the following list has been assembled. Within each global outcome, components of the outcome are alphabetized, and under each component, interventions are alphabetized.

Because many interventions are known by different names, in some places we have listed an alternate name. The possibility does exist that you know an intervention by a different name. The authors, in fact, have talked for as long as two hours about the same game under different names and not realized it. In many cases, if you are unfamiliar with an intervention, you can search the Internet and literature. This list is not exhaustive; it is a beginning compilation.

This list will help translate how drama interventions address various treatment outcomes for our colleagues in other mental and medical health fields. When they understand the "method behind our madness" (*Hamlet*, Act 2, scene 2, 193–206), they will begin to understand the value of the arts as a healing modality.

Behavioral Regulation

Anger Management

Emotion targets
Empty chair
Escalation/de-escalation of conflict
Personifying emotions (e.g., anger, flexibility, etc.)
Pop toob conversation
Postcard stories/poems variation 3
Role-play
Role reversal
Sculpting conflict

Following Directions
- Airport
- Blindfold walk (pairs)
- Blocking and rehearsing a play
- Captain is coming, the
- Elbow-to-elbow
- Go
- People-shelter-storm
- Simon says
- Taxi
- Typewriter

Impulse Control
- ABCs
- Animal transformations
- Blast-Off
- Count to 20
- Emotion orchestra/symphony
- Four corner dash
- Freeze
- Go
- Museum guard/night at the museum
- Red light, green light
- Simon says
- Sound stories
- What you think/what you say

Opposite Action Skills
- Failure celebration
- Failure vaccination
- Opposite attack
- What are you doing?
- What you think/what you say

Task Initiation and Persistence
- Embodied life maps
- Freeze and justify
- Go
- Journaling
- Maps to recovery
- Museum guard/night at the museum

- Postcard stories/poems
- Role-development with role-sort cards
- Role theatre of life
- Scene with three props/story bags
- Sculpting goals
- Self-masks
- Small group work

Task Organizational Skills

- Embodied life maps
- Fedder's Four
- Improvisation
- Maps to recovery
- Obstacle course for procrastinators/avoiders
- Relay race with no hands
- Role theatre of life
- Sculpting goals
- Self-masks
- Six-word memoirs

Cognitive Regulation

Abstract Thinking

- Balloon of addiction/illness
- Magic box
- Magic stick/tube/scarf
- Maps to recovery
- Pantomime
- Personification of emotion
- Role theatre of life
- Sculpting
- Self-masks
- Six-word memoirs
- Slow motion tug-of-war
- Story metaphor
- Symbolic thinking/metaphor
- Using scarves for costumes
- Using props

Attention Skills: Focus, Shifting

- ABCs/count to 20
- Add on memory games

Back writing
Ball throwing games (categories, questions)
Bunny-bunny
Change three
Chick-a-berry
Finding spaces
Follow the leader
Fortunately/unfortunately
Go
I challenge your story
I spy
Magic stick/tube/scarf
Mirroring
Museum guard/night at the museum
Name games
Obstacle course for procrastinators/avoiders
One-word stories
Pass your name with a movement
Pass the sound/movement
Pattern ball passing
People-shelter-storm
Postcard stories/poems variation 3
1776
Swoosh-bong
Three-ball pass
Trust circles
Who's the leader?
Word association
Yes, no, you
Zip-zap-zop

Cognitive Empathy

Body emotions
Dramatize a picture
Emotional orchestra/symphony
Empty chair
Group mood
Inside out
Personification of emotion
Postcard stories/poems
Sculpting emotions

Sharing after a psychodrama/sociodrama
Snail
Stanislavski's character development/analysis
Talk about the motives of characters in role-plays and in plays

Cognitive Flexibility

Add on memory games
Bird, beast, and fish
Empty chair
Family sculptures
Fedder's Four
Fortunately/unfortunately
Freeze and justify
Gibberish
Magic stick/tube/scarf
Name games
Pass your name with a movement
Postcard stories/poems variation 3
Scene replays
Sculpting a concept
Snail
Swoosh-bong
Winds are blowing
Yes, and

Decision Making: Evaluating and Selecting Alternatives/Solutions

Come-go-stay
Court trial
Embodied life maps
Fedder's Four
Fortunately/unfortunately
Group storytelling
Improvisation
Magic stick/tube/scarf
Maps to recovery
Museum guard/night at the museum
Postcard stories/poems variation 3
Role-development with role-sort cards
Role theatre of life
Scene replay
Scene with three props/story bags
Sculpting goals

Six-part story method
Wise mind

Define Problem

Embodied life maps
Fedder's Four
Maps to recovery
Obstacle course for procrastinators/avoiders
Playback theatre
Postcard stories/poems variation 3
Sculpting
Sculpting goals
Six-part story method
Spectrograms

Disordered Thinking (Thought Disorder)

Pass the face
Relay race with no hands
Role-development with role-sort cards
Scarf ball toss

Disorganized Thinking

Fedder's Four
Fortunately/unfortunately
Embodied life maps
Group storytelling
Maps to recovery
One-word stories
Postcard stories/poems
Psychodrama
Role-development with role-sort cards
Sculpting goals
Six-part story method
Sociodrama
Yes, no, you
Zip-zap-zop

Generate Alternatives/Solutions

Commonalities
Fedder's Four
Fortunately/unfortunately
Gibberish Dictionary
Magic scarf/magic tube
Postcard stories/poems variation 3

Relay race with no hands
Scene replay
Six-part story method
Snail
What are you doing?
Yes, and

Implement Alternatives/Solutions

Calling out emotions (and variations)
Devised theatre
Embodied life mapping
Emotion machines
Environments
Getting off the island
Improvisation
Map to recovery
Obstacle course for procrastinators
Relay race with no hands
Scenes replays
Scenes with three props

Listening Skills

ABCs/count to 20
Airport
Calling out emotions
Captain is coming, the
Court trial
Dog and bone
Drum conversations
Elbow to elbow
Emoji scenes
Finding your partner with a sound
Fortunately/unfortunately
Freeze
Freeze and justify
Group storytelling
I challenge your story
Inside out
Name games
On the bank/in the river
One-word stories
People-shelter-storm

Queen has a headache, the
Reflective listening/rephrasing
Simon says
Snail
Telephone
Three ball pass
Typewriter
Word association

Organizational Skills: Prioritizing, Goal Setting and Planning

Embodied life map
Future projection
Magic box
Map to recovery/goal
Obstacle course for procrastinators/avoiders
Playwriting and performance
Postcard stories/poems variation 3
Role-development with role-sort cards
Role theatre of life
Scene with three props/story bags
Sculpting goals
Sculpting past/present/future or continuum
Six-part story method

Problem-Solving Skills

Balloon of addiction/illness
Brainstorming for projects/plays
Embodied life mapping
Fedder's Four
Fortunately/unfortunately
Getting off the island
Hot chocolate river
Machines
Magic stick/tube/scarf
Map to recovery
Museum guard
Obstacle course for procrastinators/avoiders
Postcard stories/poems variation 3
Relay race with no hands
Scene with three props/story bags
Sculpting goals
Sculpting past/present/future or continuum

Scene replays
Six-part story method
Tangling
Who's the leader?
Yes, and

Reality Testing

Commonalities
Confronting yourself on video
Deroling
I challenge your story
Life-drama connection
Practice going in and out of dramatic reality
Role-development with role-sort cards
To tell the truth
Two truths and a lie
Wise mind

Reasoning Skills

Court trial
Embodied life maps
Fedder's Four
Freeze and justify
Guess who's guilty
I challenge your story
Map to recovery
Role-development with role-sort cards
Role theatre of life
Scene replays
Sculpting goals
Snail
To tell the truth
Two truths and a lie
Wise mind

Reframing

Change the perspective
Clams are great
Doubling
Empty chair
Fortunately/unfortunately
I challenge your story
Obstacle course for procrastinators/avoiders

Postcard stories/poems variation 3
Reframe with frame
Scene replays
Six-part story method
Snail

Self-Awareness/Reflection

Autobiographical plays/autodrama/self-revelatory performance
Balloon of addiction/illness
Body drawings
Body emotions
Check-ins and check-outs
Come-go-stay
Commonalities
Confronting yourself on video
I challenge your story
Locograms
Magic box
Obstacle course for procrastinators/avoiders
Pillow burdens
Psychiatrist
Role theatre of life
Sculpting past/present/future or continuum
Self-masks
Self-monologues
Six-word memoirs
Spectrograms
Talking to yourself in the mirror/Skyping with yourself

Sequencing

ABCs/count to 20
Add on memory games
Back writing
Bunny-bunny
Chick-a-berry
Embodied life map
Fortunately/unfortunately
Future projection
Group storytelling
Hand squeeze
Machines
Obstacle course for procrastinators/avoiders
One-word stories

Pass your name with a movement
Pattern ball passing
People-shelter-storm
Postcard stories/poems
Role-development with role-sort cards
Role theatre of life
Scene replays
Scene with three props/story bags
Sculpting goals
Sculpting past/present/future or continuum
Six-part story method
Spectrograms
Yes, no, you
Zip-zap-zop

Working Memory

Add on memory games
Bunny-bunny
Captain is coming, the
Change three
Chick-a-berry
Elbow to elbow
Fortunately/unfortunately
Go
Group storytelling
Magic stick/tube/scarf
Name games
One-word stories
Pass your name with a movement
Pattern ball passing
People-shelter-storm
Scene replays
1776
Shape copying
Swoosh-bong
Three ball pass

Emotional Regulation

Emotional Empathy

Doubling
Developmental transformations

Emotion mirroring
Emotion thermometer
Emotional spaces
Empty chair
Family sculptures
Pass the face reactions
Playback theatre
Psychodrama
Puppetry
Role reversal
Sculpting oppression
Sociodrama
Theatre of the oppressed
Witnessing

Emotion Expression

Autobiographical performance/self-revelatory performance
Calling out emotions
Developmental transformations
Emoji scenes
Emotional greetings
Emotion machine
Emotion mirroring
Emotion orchestra/symphony
Emotional spaces
Emotion targets
Emotional thermometer
Group mood
Improvisation
Inside out
Making an entrance
Pass the face
Playback theatre
Pop toob conversation
Psychodrama
Role-playing
Sculpting emotion
Sociodrama
Wise mind

Emotion Identification

Body emotions

Calling out emotions
Emoji scenes
Emotion mirroring
Emotion machine
Emotion orchestra/symphony
Emotion spectrogram
Emotion thermometer
Emotional spaces
Group mood
Inside out
Magic box
Making an entrance
Metaphorical check-ins
Obstacle course for procrastinators/avoiders
Pass the face
Personification of emotions
Postcard stories/poems
Sculpting emotions
Tone of voice exercises
Video or performance identification of triggering event

Emotion Shifting

Autobiographical therapeutic performance
Calling out emotions
Developmental transformations
Emoji scenes
Emotion mirroring
Emotional spaces
Emotional thermometer
Inside out
Magic box
Perform monologues/scenes from plays and films
Playback theatre
Psychodrama
Role-playing
Snail
Sociodrama
Wise mind

Emotional Tolerance

Autobiographical therapeutic performance
Balloon of addiction/illness

Confronting self on video
Emoji scenes
Emotion mirroring
Emotional spaces
Failure celebration
Failure vaccination
Inside out
Magic box
Making an entrance
Inside out
Perform monologues/scenes from plays and films
Sculpting a continuum
Wise mind

Identify Emotions in Self (See **Cognitive Empathy** for Identifying Emotions in Others)
Calling out emotions
Body emotions
Emoji scenes
Emotion check-ins and check-outs
Emotion sculpting
Emotion spectrogram
Emotion walk and freeze
Inside out
Magic box
Making an entrance
Pass the face reaction

Recognizing Emotional Triggers
Emotion targets
Magic box
Maps to recovery
Obstacle course for procrastinators/avoiders
Personification of emotions
Video or performance identification of triggering event

Stress Management—Coping Skills
Breathing exercises
Emotion targets
Deroling
Failure celebration
Failure vaccination
Guided fantasy
Magic box

Progressive relaxation
Wise mind

Understanding Levels of Emotional Intensity

Alba Emoting
Emotion spectrogram
Emotion thermometer
Magic shop
Making an entrance
Pass the face/body (adding to the intensity)
Personification of emotions
Sculpting a continuum
Sculpting emotions
Video or performance identification of triggering event

Locus of Control

Blindfold walks
Developmental transformations
Devised theatre
Embodied life map
Fedder's Four
Future projection
Improvisation
Line repetition
Map to recovery/goal
Magic shop
Playwriting
Psychodrama
Sculpting goals
Sculpting past/present/future or continuum
Sociodrama
Wise mind

Physiological Regulation

Body Movement Control

Airport
Animal herds
Animal transformations
Balance activities (spinning, stand up back to back, stand up front to front)
Balloons of addiction

Big/small/shape changing
Blast-off
Blindfold line
Bunny-bunny
Captain is coming, the
Chick-a-berry
Dog and bone/The Queen has a headache
Elbow to elbow
Follow the leader
Four corner dash
Games of tag
Ghost guess game
Hula hoop/bubble walk
Hula hoop pass
Machines
Mirroring
Museum guard/Night at the Museum
On the bank/in the river
Red light/green light
Shape copying
Slow motion tug of war
Snake
Splash
Tangling
Transportation
Walks: Animal/shoe/emotion/weather /environmental

Physiological Control

Drumming
Four-part breath
Guided fantasy
Mindfulness activities
Progressive relaxation

Sensory Integration/Awareness

Back writing
Balance exercises
Blast-off
Change three
Hand squeeze/pass the pulse
I spy
Imaginary tug of war

Mirroring
Pass the sound/pass the movement
Sound stories
Swoosh-bong
Walks: Animal/shoe/emotion/weather/environmental
Who's the leader?

Social-Emotional Reciprocity

Boundaries
Come-go-stay
Elbow to elbow
Finding spaces
Follow the leader
Four corner dash
Go
Going in and out of dramatic reality
Hand squeeze/pass the pulse
Hula hoop/bubble walk
In the bank/in the river
Mirroring
Machines
Pop toob conversation
Relay race with no hands
Sculpting
Snail
Tangling
Trust falls
Trust circles
Winds are blowing, the
Wise mind

Conflict Resolution
Drumming conversations
Escalation/de-escalation of conflict
Getting off the island
Line repetition
Pop toob conversation
Postcard stories/poems variation 3
Sculpting conflict
Sculpting oppression

Nonverbal Communication/Expression Skills

ABCs/count 1–20
Animal herds
Bird, beast and fish
Bunny-bunny
Come-go-stay
Drumming conversations
Environments
Gibberish
Group mood
Line repetition
Magic stick/tube/scarf
Making an entrance
Mirroring
Open scenes (tone of voice)
Pantomime games
Pass the face
Partner pantomimes
Sandtray worlds

Social Skills (engagement/interactions)

Come-go-stay
Commonalities
Devised theatre
Elbow to elbow
Emotional greetings
Improvisation
Introducing your partner
Magic stick/tube/scarf
Mirroring
Pass the face reaction
Pop toob conversation
Postcard stories/poems variation 3
Rehearsing and performing a play
Role reversal
Snail
Winds are blowing, the
Yes, and
Yes, no, you
What you think/what you say

Teamwork

Back writing
Bear, fish, mosquito
Blast-Off
Blindfold walk
Captain is coming, the
Come-go-stay
Court trial
Devised theatre
Dog and bone/the Queen has a headache
Emotional orchestra/symphony
Environments
Follow the leader
Ghost guess game
Hot chocolate river
Hula hoop pass
Imaginary magic box
Imaginary tug of war
Inside out
Machines
Mirroring
Museum guard/Night at the Museum
Pattern ball passing
People-shelter-storm
Performing a play
Playback theatre
Postcard stories/poems variation 3
Relay race with no hands
Scarf ball toss
Scene replays
Scene with three props/story bags
Sculpting
1776
Tangling
Three ball pass
Transportation
Trust carries
Trust circles
Trust falls
Who's the leader?

Word association

Trust

Airport
Blindfold walks
Finding your partner with a sound
Snail
Transportation
Trust carries
Trust circles
Trust falls

Verbal Communication/Expression Skills

Airport
Empty chair
Developmental transformations
Future projection
Gibberish
Group discussions
I challenge your story
Improvisation
Obstacle course for procrastinators/avoiders
Pop toob conversation
Reflective listening
Role-play
Sandtray story
Scene replays
Snail
Storytelling games
Telephone
Typewriter
Word association

References

Abrams, J. A., Hill, A., & Maxwell, M. (2019). Underneath the mask of the strong black woman schema: Disentangling influences of strength and self-silencing on depressive symptoms among U.S. black women. *Sex Roles, 80*(9–10), 517–526.

American Art Therapy Association. (2011). *Art therapy multicultural/diversity competencies.* Retrieved from www.arttherapy.org/upload/multiculturalcompetencies2011.pdf

American Psychiatric Association. (2013). *Diagnostic and statistical manual of mental disorders* (5th ed.).

American Psychological Association. (2017). *Multicultural guidelines: An ecological approach to context, identity, and intersectionality, 2017.* https://www.apa.org/about/policy/multicultural-guidelines.

Americans with Disabilities Act of 1990. §42 U.S.C. 12101 et seq. (1990). https://www.ada.gov/pubs/adastatute08.htm

Armstrong, C. R., Rozenberg, M., Powell, M. A., Honce, J., Bronstein, L., Gingras, G., & Han, E. (2016). A step toward empirical evidence: Operationalizing and uncovering drama therapy change processes. *The Arts in Psychotherapy, 49*, 27–33. https:// doi.org/10.1016/j.aip.2016.05.007

Bailey, S. (1999). *What is drama therapy*? Retrieved from www.dramatherapycentral.com/What-is-drama-therapy/

Bailey, S. (2009). Performance in drama therapy. In D. R. Johnson & R. Emunah (Eds.), *Current approaches in drama therapy* (2nd ed., pp. 374–392). Charles C. Thomas.

Bailey, S. (2010). *Barrier-free theatre: Including everyone in theatre arts—in schools, recreation and arts programs—regardless of (dis)ability.* Idyll Arbor.

Bailey, S., & Dickinson, P. (2016). The importance of safely de-roling. *Methods: A Journal of Acting Pedagogy, 2*, 1–18.

Bailey, S., & Dickinson, P. (2018). Teaching beyond the traditional: Generating ethics and social justice in applied theatre curricula. In A. Fliotis & G. Medford (Eds.) *New directions in teaching theatre arts* (pp. 225–248). Palgrave MacMillan. https://doi.org/10.1007/978-3-319-89767-7.

Baker, L., & Brown, A. L. (1984). Metacognitive skills and reading. In P. D. Pearson, R. Barr, M. L. Kamil, & P. Mosenthal (Eds.), *Handbook of reading research* (Vol. 1, pp. 353–394). Routledge.

Barr, A. F., Jr. (1980). *Picasso: Fifty years of his art.* Arno Press.

Bell, C. C., Dixie-Bell, D. D., & Thompson, B. (1986). Further studies on the prevalence of isolated sleep paralysis in black subjects. *Journal of the National Medical Association, 78*(7), 649–659.

Blatner, A., & Blatner, A. (1988). *The art of play.* Springer.

Bloch, S. (1993). Alba Emoting: A psycho-physiological technique to help actors create and control real emotions. *Theatre Topics, 3*(2), 121–138.

Boal, A. (1992). *Games for actors and nonactors.* Theatre Communications Group.

Boal, A. (1993). *Theatre of the oppressed.* Theatre Communications Group.

Boal, A. (1995). *The rainbow of desire.* Routledge.

Bodrova, E., Germeroth, C., & Leong, D. J. (2013). Play and self-regulation: Lessons from Vygotsky. *American Journal of Play, 6*(1), 111–123.

Bodrova, E., & Leong, D. J. (2007). *Tools of the mind: The Vygotskian approach to early childhood education* (2nd ed.). Pearson/Merrill Prentice Hall.

Bornmann, B. A., Mitelman, S. A., & Beer, D. A. (2007). Psychotherapeutic relaxation: How it relates to levels of aggression in a school within inpatient child psychiatry: A pilot study. *The Arts in Psychotherapy, 37*, 216–222. https://doi.org/10.1016/j.aip.2007.01.004

Brammer, L. M., & MacDonald, G. (2003). *The helping relationship: Process and skills* (8th ed.). Prentice-Hall.

Braniecka, A., Hanc, M., Wotkowicz, I., Chrzczonowicz-Stepien, A., Mikotajonek, A. & Lipiec, M. (2018). Is it worth turning a trigger into a joke? Humor as an emotion regulation strategy in remitted depression. *Brain and Behavior.* https://doi.org/10.1002/brb3.1213

British Association of Dramatherapy Equity and Diversity SubCommittee (n.d.). https://badth.org.uk

Brown, S., & Vaughn, C. (2009). *Play: How it shapes the brain, opens the imagination, and invigorates the soul.* Avery.

Canadian Association for Music Therapy. (1999). *Canadian association for music therapy: Code of ethics.* https://www.musictherapy.ca/about-camt-music-therapy/camt-ethics/

Carnerio, E. M., Barbosa, L. P., Marson, J. M., Alves Terra J., Jr., Martins, C. J., Modesto, D., de Resende, L. A., & Borges, M. (2017). Effectiveness of spiritist "passe" for anxiety levels, depression, pain, muscle tension, well-being, and physiological parameters in cardiovascular inpatients: A randomized controlled trial. *Complementary Therapies in Medicine, 30*, 73–78. https://doi.org/10.1016/j.ctim.2016.11.008

Cassidy, S., Gumley, A., & Turnbull, S. (2017). Safety, play, enablement and active involvement: Themes from a grounded theory study of practitioner and client experiences of change processes in dramatherapy. *The Arts in Psychotherapy, 55*, 174–185. https://doi.org/10.1016/j.aip.2017.05.007

Casson, J. (2004). *Drama, psychotherapy and psychosis: Dramatherapy and psychodrama with people who hear voices.* Brunner-Routledge.

Cattanach, A. (1994). Dramatic play with children. In S. Jennings, A. Cattanach, S. Mitchell, A. Chesner, & B. Meldrum (Eds.), *The handbook of drama therapy* (pp. 133–144). Routledge.

Ceunen, E., Vlaeyen, J. W. S., & Van Diest, I. (2016). On the origin of interoception. *Frontiers in Psychology, 7*, 743. https://doi.org/10.3389/fpsyg.2016.00743

Chaiklin, S., & Wengrower, H. (2015). *The art and science of dance/movement therapy.* Routledge.

Chapman, E. J. (2014). Using dramatic reality to reduce depressive symptoms: A qualitative study. *The Arts in Psychotherapy, 41*(2), 137–144.

Chekov, M. (1991). *On the technique of acting.* HarperCollins.

Coholic, D., Fraser, M., Robinson, B., & Lougheed, S. (2012). Promoting resilience within child protection: The suitability of arts-based and experiential group programs for children in care. *Social Work in Groups, 35*(4), 345–361.

Corkin, S. (2013). *Permanent present tense: The unforgettable life of the amnesic patient, H.M.* Basic Books.

Cowan, N. (2008). What are the differences between long term, short term, and working memory? *Progress in Brain Research, 169*, 323–338. https://doi.org/10.1016/S0079-6123(07)00020-9

Csikszentmihalyi, M. (1990). *Flow: The psychology of optimal experience.* Harper & Row.

Csikszentmihalyi, M. (1996). *Creativity: Flow and the psychology of discovery and invention.* HarperCollins.

Damasio, A. (1994). *Descartes' error: Emotion, reason and the human brain.* Avon.

Damasio, A. (1999). *The feeling of what happens.* Harcourt.

Davidson, L., Shahar, G., Lawless, M. S., Sells, D., & Tondora, J. (2006, Summer). Play, pleasure, and other positive life events: "Non-specific" factors in recovery from mental illness? *Psychiatry, 69*(2), 151–163.

Dickinson, P. E., Schwartzmueller, A., & Martin, B. (2014). An empirical assessment of an activity to teach sensory change in aging. *Teaching of Psychology, 41*(3), 242–245.

Doidge, N. (2007). *The brain that changes itself: Stories of personal triumph from the frontiers of brain science.* Viking.

Downs, W. M., & Russin, R. U. (2004). *Naked playwriting: The art, the craft, and the life laid bare.* Silman-James Press.

Duell, O. K. (1994). Extended wait time and university students' achievements. *American Educational Research Journal, 31*(2), 397–414.

Duggan, M., & Grainger, R. (1997). *Imagination, identification and catharsis in theatre and therapy.* Jessica Kingsley.

Education Amendments Act of 1972, 20 U.S.C. §§1681 – 1688 (2018).

EEOC (United States Equal Employment Opportunity Commission). (2002). *Enforcement guidance: Reasonable accommodation and undue hardship under the Americans with Disabilities Act.* https://www.eeoc.gov/policy/docs/accommodation.html

Egan, G. (2013). *The skilled helper: A problem management and opportunity-development approach to helping* (10th ed.). Brooks/Cole.

Elkind, D. (1967). Egocentrism in adolescence, *Child Development, 38*, 1025–1034.

Emunah, R. (2020). *Acting for real: Drama therapy process, technique, and performance* (2nd ed.). Routledge.

Emunah, R., & Johnson, D. R. (Eds.). (2009). *Current approaches in drama therapy* (2nd ed.). Charles C. Thomas.

Family Education Rights and Privacy Act of 1974. 20 U.S.C. § 1232g; 34 CFR Part 99.

Felton, G. S., & Biggs, B. E. (1972). Teaching internalization behavior to collegiate low achievers in group psychotherapy. *Psychotherapy, 9*(3), 281–283.

Fershleiser, R., & Smith, L. (2008). *Not quite what I was planning: Six-word memoirs by writers famous & obscure*. HarperCollins.

Flavel, J. H. (1963). *The developmental psychology of Jean Piaget*. D. Van Nostrad.

Foulds, M. L. (1971). Changes in locus of internal-external control: A growth experience. *Comparative Group Studies, 2*(3), 293–300.

Gaebel, W. (2015). ICD-11 and DSM-5-Similarities and differences. *European Psychiatry: The Journal of the European Psychiatric Association, 30*, 115. https://doi.org/10.1016/S0924-9338(15)31836–8

Gallagher, H. L., & Frith, C. (2003). Functional imaging of "theory of mind." *Trends in Cognitive Sciences, 7*(2), 77–83.

Gallaudet University (2015). *American Deaf culture*. Retrieved from https://www3.gallaudet.edu/clerc-center/info-to-go/deaf-culture/american-deaf-culture.html

Gallese, V. (2016). Finding the body in the brain. In B. P. McLaughlin & H. Kornblith (Eds.). *Goldman and his critics*. John Wiley. https://doi.org/ 10.1002/9781118609378.ch14

Gallese, V., & Cuccio, V. (2018). The neural exploitation hypothesis and its implications for an embodied approach to language and cognition: Insights from the study of action verbs processing and motor disorders in Parkinson's disease. *Cortex, 100*, 215–225. https://doi.org/10.1016/j.cortex.2018.01.010

Gallese, V., Kesers, C., & Rizzolatti, G. (2004). A unifying view of the basis of social cognition. *Trends in Cognitive Sciences, 8*(9), 396–403. https://doi.org/10.1016/j.tics.2004.07.002

Gallese, V., & Lakoff, G. (2005). The brain's concepts: The role of the sensory-motor system in conceptual knowledge. *Cognitive Neuroscience, 22*(3/4), 455–479.

Gilovich, T., Medvec, V., & Savitsky, K. (2000). The spotlight effect in social judgement: An egocentric bias in estimates of the salience of one's own actions and appearance. *Journal of Personality and Social Psychology, 78*(2), 211–222.

Glennie, E. (2003, February). *How to truly listen*. [Videofile]. Retrieved from https://www.ted.com/talks/evelyn_glennie_shows_how_to_listen#t-967130

Gioia, G. A., Isquith, P. K., Retzlaff, P. D., & Espy, K. A. (2002). Confirmatory factor analysis of the Behavior Rating Inventory of Executive Function (BRIEF) in a clinical sample. *Child Neuropsychology, 8*(4), 249–257.

Goldberg, E. (2009). *The new executive brain: Frontal lobes in a complex world.* Oxford University Press.

Goosby, B. J., & Heidbrink, C. (2013). The transgenerational consequences of discrimination on African-American health outcomes. *Sociology Compass, 7*, 630–643. https://doi.org/ 10.1111/soc4.12054

Grainger, R. (2008). Dramatherapy and cognitive readjustment. *Counseling Psychology Review, 23*(3), 40–46.

Grant, A. M. (2001). Rethinking psychological mindedness: Metacognition, self-reflection, and insight. *Behaviour Change, 18*(1), 8–17.

Greenberg, G. (2013). *The book of woe: The DSM and the unmaking of psychiatry.* Blue Rider Press.

Greene, M. C., & Carpenter, J. M. (2011). Transporting into narrative worlds: New directions for the scientific study of literature. *Scientific Study of Literature, 1*(1), 113–122.

Gross, J. J. (1998). Antecedent- and response-focused emotion regulation: Divergent consequences for experience, expression, and physiology. *Journal of Personality and Social Psychology, 74*, 224–237.

Hamamci, Z. (2006). Integrating psychodrama and cognitive behavioral therapy to treat moderate depression. *The Arts in Psychotherapy, 33*, 199–207. https://doi.org/ 10.1016/j.aip.2006.02.001

Harris, J. (2009). The evolutionary neurobiology, emergence and facilitation of empathy. In T. F. D. Farrow & P. W. R. Woodruff (Eds.), *Empathy in Mental Illness* (pp. 168–186). Cambridge University Press.

Hartford, M. E. (1972). *Groups in social work: Application of small group theory and research to social work practice.* Columbia University Press.

Health Insurance Portability and Accountability Act of 1996. Pub. L. No. 104–191, § 264, 110 Stat.1936.

Hearing Link (n.d.). *Cochlear implants.* https://www.hearinglink.org/ your-hearing/implants/ cochlear-implants/

Hendricks, M. A., & Buchanan, T. W. (2016). Individual differences in cognitive control processes and their relationship to emotion regulation. *Cognition and Emotion, 30*, 912–924. https://doi.org/10.1080/02699931.2015.1032893

Heise, D. (2014, May). Steeling and resilience. *Art Education, 67*, 26–30. https://doi.org/ 10.1080/00043125.2014.11519270

Hermann, J. (1992). *Trauma and recovery.* HarperCollins.

Hoffower, K. (2018). *Strength-based drama therapy with groups.* Independently published.

Hook, J. N., Davis, D. E., Owen, J., Worthington, E. L., Jr., & Utsey, S. O. (2013). Cultural humility: Measuring openness to culturally diverse clients. *Journal of Counseling Psychology, 60*(3), 353–366.

Hynes, M. J. (2018, August 1). Kids need play and recess. Their mental health may depend on it. http://blogs.edweek.org/edweek/finding_common_ground/2018/08/the_existential_mental_health_crisis_in_k-12_education_the_need_for_play_and_recess.html

Iacoboni, M., Molnar-Szakacs, I., Gallese, V., Buccino, G., Mazziotta, J. C., & Rizzolatti, G. (2005). Grasping the intentions of others in one's own mirror neuron system. *PLOS Biology, 3*(3), 529–535.

Ibrahim, F. A., Dinsmore, J. A., Estrada, D., & D'Andrea, M. (2011). The counselors for social justice (CSJ) code of ethics. *Journal for Social Action in Counseling and Psychology, 3*(2), 1–21. https://jsacp.tumblr.com

Jennings, S. (1998). *Introduction to dramatherapy: Theatre and healing—Ariadne's ball of thread.* Jessica Kingsley.

Johnson, C. D., Benson, P. V., & Seaton, J. B. (1997). *Educational audiology handbook.* Singular Publishing Group.

Johnson, D. R. (1991). The theory and technique of transformations in drama therapy. *The Arts in Psychotherapy, 18*(4), 285–300.

Johnson, D. R. (2009). Emotional attention set-shifting and its relationship to anxiety and emotion regulation. *Journal of Emotion, 9*, 681–690. https://doi.org/10.1037/a0017095

Jones, P. (1996). *Drama as therapy: Theatre as living.* Jessica Kingsley.

Jones, P. (2007). *Drama as therapy: Theory, practice and research* (2nd ed.). Jessica Kingsley.

Keisari, S., & Palgi, Y. (2017). Life-crossroads on stage: Integrating life-review and drama therapy for older adults. *Aging & Mental Health, 20*(10), 1079–1089.

Kidder, R. M. (2009). *How good people make tough choices: Resolving the dilemmas of ethical living.* HarperPerennial.

Kiefer, M., & Trumpp, N. M. (2012). Embodiment theory and education: The foundations of cognition in perception and action. *Trends in Neuroscience and Education, 1*(1), 15–20.

Kilgore, T. (2019). Exploring the cochlear implant controversy: The role of and experience with Deaf culture for parents of pediatric cochlear implant users. *Ursidae: The Undergraduate Research Journal at the University of Northern Colorado, 5*(2), Article 4.

King, J. L. (Ed.). (2016). *Art therapy, trauma, and neuroscience: Theoretical and practical perspectives.* Routledge.

Kipper, D. A., Davelaar, P. S., & Herst, S. (2009). The relationship between spontaneity and inhibition. *The Arts in Psychotherapy, 36*(5), 329–334.

Klein, G. (2013). *Seeing what others don't: The remarkable ways we gain insight.* Public Affairs.

Kruger, J., & Dunning, D. (1999). Unskilled and unaware of it: How difficulties in recognizing one's own incompetence lead to inflated self-assessments. *Journal of Personality and Social Psychology, 77*(6), 1121–1134.

Krznaric, R. (2014). *Empathy: Why it matters, and how to get it.* Perigee.

Lahad, M. (1992). Story-making in assessment method for coping with stress: Six-piece storymakingand BASIC Ph. In S. Jennings (Ed.), *Dramatherapy theory and practice 2* (pp. 150–163). Routledge.

Lahad, M., Shacham, M., & Ayalon, O. (2013). *The "BASIC-PH" model of coping and resiliency—Theory, research, and cross-cultural application.* Jessica Kingsley.

Landy, R. J. (1991). The drama therapy role method. *Dramatherapy, 14*(2), 7–15. https://doi.org/10.1080/02630672.1992.9689810

Landy, R. J. (1993). *Persona and performance.* Guilford Press.

Landy, R. J. (2009). Role theory and the role method of drama therapy. In D. R. Johnson & R. Emunah (Eds.), *Current approaches in drama therapy* (2nd ed., pp. 65–88). Charles C. Thomas.

Lanzoni, S. (2018). *Empathy: A history.* Yale University Press.

Levitin, D. L. (2008). *The world in six songs: How the musical brain created human nature.* Dutton.

Lewis, P., & Johnson, D. R. (Eds.). (2000). *Current approaches to drama therapy.* Charles C. Thomas.

Linehan, M. (1993). *Cognitive-Behavioral treatment of borderline personality disorder.* Guilford Press.

Lusseyran, J. (1994). Poetry in Buchenwald. In L. E. Sullivan (Ed.), *The parabola book of healing* (pp. 5–16). Continuum.

Ma, R., Mann, F., Wang, J., Lloyd-Evans, B., Terhune, J., Al-Shihabi, A., & Johnson, S. (2019). The effectiveness of interventions for reducing subjective and objective social isolation among people with mental health problems: A systematic review. *Social Psychiatry and Psychiatric Epidemiology: The International Journal for Research in Social and Genetic Epidemiology and Mental Health Services*, 1-38. https://doi.org/10.1007/s00127-019-01800-z

Marich, J., & Daniger, S. (2017). *EMDR therapy and mindfulness for trauma-focused care.* Springer.

Marlatt, G. A., & Marques, J. K. (1976, March). Meditation, self-control and alcohol use. Paper presented at the Banff International Conference on Behavior Modification.

McLaren, K. (2013). *The art of empathy: A complete guide to life's most essential skill.* Sounds True.

Mehdi, P. R., Sen, A. K., & Sen Mazumdar, D. P. (1997). The usefulness of psychodrama in treating depressed patients. *Indian Journal of Clinical Psychology, 24*(1), 82–92.

Mehdi, P. R., Sen Mazumdar, D. P., & Sen, A. K. (1997). The effectiveness of psychodrama in changing attitudes among depressed patients. *Journal of Personality and Clinical Studies, 13*(1–2), 19–23.

Miller, G. A., Galanter, E., & Pribram, K. H. (1960). *Plans and the structure of behavior.* Henry Holt.

Miller, S. D., Duncan, B. L., & Hubble, M. A. (1997). *Escape from Babel: Toward a unifying language for psychotherapy practice.* W. W. Norton.

Moore, R. C., Straus, E., Dev, S. I., Parish, S. M., Sueko, S., & Eiler, L. T. (2017). Development and pilot of randomized control trial of a drama program to enhance well-being among older adults. *The Arts in Psychotherapy, 52*, 1–9. https://doi.org/10.1016/j.aip.2016.09.007

Moreno, J. L. (1959). *Psychodrama* (Vols. 1 & 2). Beacon House.

Moreno, J. L. (1987). Spontaneity and catharsis. In J. Fox (Ed.), *The essential Moreno: Writings on Psychodrama, group method, and spontaneity by J.L. Moreno, M.D* (pp. 41–62). Springer.

Moreno, J. L. (1993). *Who shall survive? Foundations of Sociometry, Group Psychotherapy, and Sociodrama* (student edition). American Society for Group Psychotherapy and Psychodrama.

Najdowski, A.C., Persicke, A., & Kung, E. (2014). Executive Functions. In E. Graneesheh, J. Tarbos, A. C. Najbowski, & J. Kornack (Eds.), *Evidence-based treatment for children with autism: The CARD model* (pp. 356–389). Elsevier.

National Association of the Deaf (2003). *Position statement on mental health services for people who are Deaf and hard of hearing (2003): Open letter to the mental health community and allied service providers.* https://www.nad.org/about-us/position-statements/position-statement-on-mental-health-services/

National Association of the Deaf (NAD) (2019a). *What is NAD's position on cochlear implants?* https://www.nad.org/about-us/faq/

National Association of the Deaf (NAD) (2019b). *I am a service provider. Do I need to provide and pay for interpreter services for a deaf or hard of hearing client/patient?* https://www.nad.org/about-us/law-advocacy-center/faq/

National Cued Speech Organization (n.d.). *Definition of cued speech.* http://www.cuedspeech.org/cued-speech-definition

National Endowment for the Arts (2005). *Design for accessibility: A cultural administrator's handbook.* https://www.arts.gov/sites/default/files/Design-for-Accessibility.pdf

National Endowment for the Arts (2013). *The arts and humanities accessibility checklist.* https://www.arts.gov/publications/arts-and-humanities-accessibility-checklist

National Research Council (2000). *How people learn: Brain, mind, experience, and school, (expanded edition).* The National Academies Press. https://doi.org/10.17226/9853

Niedenthal, P. M. (2007). Embodying emotion. *Science, 361*(5827), 1002–1005.

North American Drama Therapy Association (2015). Guidelines on Cultural Response/ability in Training, Research, Practice, Supervision, Advocacy and Organizational Change. https://www.nadta.org/about-nadta/diversity/Cultural_Responsibility_Guidelines

North American Drama Therapy Association (NADTA) (2019a). NADTA Code, Ethical Principles. https://www.nadta.org/assets/documents/updated-nadta-code-of-ethics-2019.pdf

North American Drama Therapy Association (NADTA) (2019b). Resources. https://www.nadta.org/what-is-drama-therapy/Resources.html

Northen, H. (1969). *Social work with groups.* Columbia University Press.

Nowicki, S. (2016). *Choice or chance: Understanding your locus of control and why it matters.* Prometheus Books.

Nummenmaa, L., Hirvonen, J., Parkkola, R., & Hietanen, J. K. (2008). Is emotional contagion special? An Fmri study on neural systems for affective and cognitive empathy. *NeuroImage, 43*(3), 571–580.

Nuwer, R. (2013). There are 58 versions of Little Red Riding Hood, Some 1,000 years older than the brothers Grimms. *Smithsonian Magazine*. https://www.smithsonianmag.com/smart-news/there-are-58-versions-of-little-red-riding-hood-some-1000-years-older-than-the-brothers-grimms-180947704/#GTAcOjy882SYario.99

Okun, B. F., & Kantrowitz, R. E. (2015). *Effective helping: Interviewing and counseling techniques* (8th ed.). Cengage Learning.

O'Leary, M. R., Donovan, D. M., Hague, W. H., & Shea, R. (1975). Shifts in component factors of locus of control as a function of treatment in male alcoholics. *Journal of Clinical Psychology, 31(2)*, 359–361.

O'Leary, M. R., Donovan, D. M., & O'Leary, D. E. (1976). Changes in perceived and experienced control among inpatient alcoholics. *Journal of Clinical Psychology, 32*(2), 500–504.

Ornstein, A. (2006). Artistic creativity and the healing process. *Psychoanalytic Inquiry, 26*(3), 386–406.

Ophir, E., Nass, C., & Wagner, A. D. (2009). Cognitive control in media multitaskers. *Proceedings of the National Academy of Sciences of the United States of America, Vol. 106*, 15583–15587. https://doi.org/10.1074/pnas.0903620106

Oziel, L. J., & Orbitz, F. W. (1975). Control orientation in alcoholics related to extent of treatment. *Journal of Studies on Alcohol, 36*(1), 158–161.

Pattison, E. J. (1973). Effects of touch on self-exploration and the therapeutic relationship. *Journal of Consulting and Clinical Psychology, 40*(2), 170–175.

Pellis, S. M., Pellis, V. C., & Himmler, B. T. (2014). How play makes for a more adaptive brain: A comparative and neural perspective. *American Journal of Play, 7*(1), 73–98.

Pendzik, S. (2003). Six keys for assessment in drama therapy. *The Arts in Psychotherapy, 30*(2), 91–99.

Pendzik, S. (2006). On dramatic reality and its therapeutic function in drama therapy. *The Arts in Psychotherapy, 33*(4), 271–280.

Pendzik, S. (2008). Using the 6-Key Model as an intervention tool in drama therapy. *The Arts in Psychotherapy, 35*(5), 340–354.

Pendzik, S. (2012). The 6-key model—An integrative assessment approach. In D. R. Johnson, S. Pendzik, & S. Snow (Eds.), *Assessment in drama therapy* (pp. 197–222). Charles C. Thomas.

Pendzik, S. (2018). Drama therapy and the invisible realm. *Drama Therapy Review, 4*(2), 183–197.

Pendzik, S., Emunah, R., & Johnson, D. R. (2016). *The self in performance: Autobiographical, self-revelatory, and authoethnographic forms of therapeutic theatre*. Palgrave Macmillan.

Pennycook, G., Ross, R. M., Koehler, D. J., & Fugelsang, J. A. (2017). Dunning-Kruger effects and reasoning: Theoretical implications of the failure to recognize incompetence. *Psychonomic Bulletin and Review, 24*, 1774–1784. https://doi.org/10.3758/s13423-017-1242-7

Peterson, C. (2006). *A primer in positive psychology*. Oxford University Press.

Phillips, M. E. (1994). The use of drama and puppetry in occupational therapy during the 1920's and 1930's. *The American Journal of Occupational Therapy, 50*(3), 229–233.

Prentki, T. (2016). *Applied theatre: Development*. London, UK: Bloomsbury Methuen Drama.

Raniszewska-Wyrwa, A. (2014). The ethics of touch: Ethical aspects of using touch in therapeutic practice. *Studia Philosophiae Christianae, 50*(2), 85–104.

Rotter, J. B. (1966). Generalized expectancies for internal versus external control of reinforcement. *Psychological Monographs: General and Applied*, *80*, 1–28. https://doi.org/10.1037/h0092976

Rowe, M. B. (1986). Wait time: Slowing down may be a way of speeding up. *Journal of Teacher Education, 37*(1), 43–50.

Rubin, S. (2008). Women, food, and feelings: Drama therapy with women who have eating disorders. In S. L. Brooke (Ed.), *The creative therapies and eating disorders* (pp. 173–193). Charles C. Thomas.

Rubin, S. (2015). Almost magic: Working with the shame that underlies depression: Using drama therapy in the imaginal realm. In S. L. Brooke & C. E. Myers (Eds.), *The use of the creative therapies in treating depression* (pp. 231–244). Charles C. Thomas.

Sajnani, N., & Johnson, D. R. (Eds.). (2014) *Trauma-informed drama therapy: Transforming clinics, classrooms and communities*. Charles C. Thomas.

Saldana, J. (2016). *Ethnotheatre: From page to stage*. Routledge.

Sawyer, R. K. (2006). *Explaining creativity: The science of human innovation*. Oxford University Press.

Schaefer, S. (2018). Embodiment helps children solve a spatial working memory task: Interactions with age and gender. *Journal of Cognitive Enhancement,* 1–12. https://doi.org/10.1007/s41465-018-0081-4

Scheff, T. J. (1979). *Catharsis in healing, ritual, and drama*. iUniverse.com.

Schraw, G., & Moshman, D. (1995). Metacognitive theories. *Educational Psychology Review*, *7*(4), 351–371.

Seligman, M. E. P. (1991). *Learned optimism: How to change your mind and your life*. Alfred A. Knopf.

Seligman, M. E. P. (2002). *Authentic happiness: Using the new positive psychology to realize your potential for lasting fulfillment*. Free Press.

Seligman, M. E. P. (2011). *Flourish: A visionary new understanding of happiness and well-being*. Free Press.

Shafer, P. O., & Dean, P. M. (2018). *Vagus nerve stimulation (VNS)*. https://www.epilepsy.com/learn/treating-seizures-and-epilepsy/devices/vagus-nerve-stimulation-vns

Shakespeare, W. (1992). *Hamlet: Prince of Denmark. Folger Shakespeare Library, Updated Edition*. Simon & Schuster.

Shamay-Tsoory, S. G., Aharon-Peretz, J., & Perry, D. (2009). Two systems for empathy: A double dissociation between emotional and cognitive empathy in inferior frontal gyrus versus ventromedial prefrontal lesions. *Brain: A Journal of Neurology*. http://brain.oxfordjournals. https://doi.org/10.1093/brain/awn279

Shapiro, F., & Forrest, M. S. (2004). *EMDR: Eye movement desensitization and eyeprocessing* (updated ed.). Perseus Books.

Siegel, D. J. (1999). *The developing mind: How relationships and the brain interact to shape who we are*. Guilford Press.

Sowden, P. T., Clements, L., Redlich, C., & Lewis, C. (2015). Improvisation facilitates divergent thinking and creativity: Realizing a benefit of primary school arts education. *Psychology of Aesthetics, Creativity, and the Arts, 9*, 128–138. https://doi.org/10.1037/aca0000018

Spandler, H., Secker, J., Kent, L., Hacking, S., & Shenton, J. (2007). Catching life: The contribution of arts initiatives to recovery approaches in mental health. *Journal of Psychiatric and Mental Health Nursing, 14*(8), 791–799.

Spinka, M. Newberry, R. C., & Bekoff, M. (2001). Mammalian play: Training for the unexpected. *Quarterly Review of Biology, 76*(2), 141–168.

Spolin, V. (1963). *Improvisation for the theatre: A handbook of teaching and directing techniques*. Northwestern University Press.

Stanislavsky, C. (1948). *An actor prepares*. Theatre Arts Books.

Staub, E. (1987). Commentary on part 1. In N. Eisenberg & J. Strayer (Eds.), *Empathy and its development* (pp. 103–115). Cambridge University Press.

Stein, K. (2007). *The genius engine: Where memory, reason, passion, violence and creativity intersect in the human brain*. John Wiley.

Stuckey, H. L., & Nobel, J. (2010). The connection between art, healing, and public health: A review of current literature. *American Journal of Public Health, 100*(2), 254–263.

Tehrani, J. J. (2013). The phylogeny of little red riding hood. *PLoS ONE, 8*(11), e78871. https://doi.org/10.1371/journal.kone.0078871

Terzioglu, C., & Ozkano, B. (2018). Psychodrama and the emotional state of women dealing with infertility. *Sexuality and Disability, 36*, 87–99. https://doi.org/10.1007/s11195-017-9514-8

Tuckman, B. W. (1965). Developmental sequence in small groups. *Psychological Bulletin, 63*(6), 384–399.

van der Kolk, B. (2014). *The body keeps the score: Brain, mind, and body in the healing of trauma*. Viking.

Van Lith, T., Fenner, P., & Schofield, M. (2010). The lived experience of art making as a companion to the mental health recovery process. *Disability and Rehabilitation, 33*(8), 652–660.

Vernig, P. M. (2011). Family roles in homes with alcohol-dependent parents: An evidenced-based review. *Substance Abuse and Misuse, 46*, 535–542. https://doi.org/10.3109/10826084.2010.501676

Voegler, C., & Montez, M. (2007). *The writer's journey: Mythic structure for writers* (3rd ed.). Michael Wiese Productions.

Volkas, A. (2009). Healing the wounds of history: Drama therapy in collective trauma and intercultural conflict resolution. In D. R. Johnson & R. Emunah (Eds.), *Current approaches in drama therapy* (2nd ed., pp. 145–171). Charles C. Thomas.

Vygotsky, L. (1978). *Mind in society: The development of higher psychological processes*. Harvard University Press.

Wegscheider, S. (1981). *Another chance: Hope and health for the alcoholic family*. Science and Behavior Books.

Weininger, O. (1988). "What If" and "As If": Imagination and pretend play in early childhood. In K. Egan & D. Nadaner, (Eds.), *Imagination and education* (pp. 141–152). Columbia University: Teacher's College Press.

Williams, K. D. (2011, January/February). The pain of exclusion. *Scientific American Mind*, 21(6), 30–37.

Winnicott, D. W. (1990). *Playing and reality*. Routledge.

World Health Organization (2018a) *Classifications*. https://www.WHO.int/classifications/ICD/en/

World Health Organization (2018b). *ICD-11 for mortality and morbidity statistics*. https://ICD.WHO.int/browse11/l-m/en

World Health Organization (2018c). *Mental health*. https://www.WHO.int/mental_health/management/en/

Yalom, I., & Leszcz, M. (2005). *The theory and practice of group psychotherapy* (5th ed.). Basic Books.

Index

1776 166, 228, 235, 243

A

abstract thinking 49, 110, 124, 151, 164–165, 211, 218, 227
accommodation vii, xvi, 51, 145–146, 150–174, 198, 217–219
ACOA, *see* adult children of alcoholics
active witnessing xv, 24, 32
ADA, *see* Americans with disabilties act
adaptation vii, xvi, 9, 114, 145–146, 150–174, 217–219
ADHD, *see* Attention Deficit Hyperactivity Disorder
adult children of alcoholics 185
aesthetic distance 30–32, 38, 100, 105, 107, 109, 110, 202, 209, 211
aging simulation 27–28
alexithymia 58, 67
allergies 162
altruism 9, 10–11
Americans with disabilities act (ADA) 157, 160, 172
American sign language (ASL) 147, 159, 160
archetypes xii, 126
as if 16, 21, 24, 29
aside 38
ASL, *see* American sign language
ATP, *see* autobiographical therapeutic performance
attention, *see* executive functioning
attention deficit hyperactivity disorder (ADHD) 25, 50, 51, 55, 115, 166–167, 199
attention-seeking behavior 7, 14, 107, 200, 209
autobiographical therapeutic performance 189–190

B

Bailey, Sally iii, xi, xv, xvi, 6, 12, 18, 21, 33, 34, 38, 57, 59, 119, 157
bang! 104, 117, 177
back-writing 166, 228, 234, 240, 243
blast-off 111, 120, 226, 240, 243
blind, *see* visual impairment
blindfold walk 99, 226, 239, 243, 244
Boal, Augusto xiii, 21
bunny bunny 170, 228, 234, 235, 240, 242

C

calling out emotions 62, 231, 236, 237, 238
captain is coming, the 166, 226, 231, 235, 240, 243
Casson, John 67
catharsis 9, 14, 18, 33
check-in 61, 81, 115–116, 118, 164, 186, 189, 213, 221, 234, 237, 238
change three 55, 228, 235, 240
chick-a-berry 170, 228, 234, 235, 240

children 43, 49, 65
and development 15, 59, 170
and FERPA 187–188
and locus of control 68–70
and play xiii, 16, 23–28
and ritual 115
and imagination 28, 124
and metacognition 112, 212
and puppets 153
and cochlear implants 160
and language comprehension 169–170
civil rights 179–180, 220
closure xv, 9, 12, 19, 92, 109, 111, 115, 118–121, 167, 211, 213–214
cochlear implant vii, 158–160, 161, 219
cognitive reappraisal 62
concentration 48, 56, 137, 139
concrete communication xi, 7, 100, 107, 109, 110, 148, 165, 170, 211, 216
concrete objects/experiences 24, 28, 49, 60, 100, 108, 121, 124, 132, 151, 153, 164, 165, 167, 171, 200, 210, 218
concrete thinking 164–165, 170
core concepts of drama therapy xvi, 21, 24–33
core concepts of group development 05–Jan
stage one: orientation 07–Jun
stage two: conflict 7–8, 17
stage three: cohesiveness 7, 8, 138, 140
stage four: working 8, 140
stage five: terminatio 09–Aug
corrective recapitulation of the primary family group 9, 11
counterrole 135
creativity 16, 45–49, 71
big c, little c 47–48
preparatio 46–48
incubation 46–47
insight x, 46–49
verification 46–47
evaluation 46
elaboration 46, 48
Csikszentmihalyi, Mihalyi 42, 50
cued speech 159
cultural appropriation 150, 152–155, 179, 180–181, 216–217, 220
cultural aspects of diagnosis 82
cultural competency xvi, 146–156, 175, 182
cultural humility xvi, 148–149, 154–155, 174

D

Deaf/deaf vii, 147, 151, 158–161, 172, 218
Deaf culture vii, 147, 159
defensive 7
deficit-based 39, 42–45, 76–77, 89–91
dementia 112, 124, 166–168, 171, 212
Alzheimer's disease 124, 166, 168, 171
Huntington's disease 166
Parkinson's disease 166
deroling 23–24, 27, 35, 59, 95, 118–121, 137, 167, 214, 233, 238
developmental transformations 32, 33, 35, 114, 120, 177, 180, 184, 199, 235, 236, 237, 239, 244
devising a play xv, 184, 189
diabetes 27, 86, 161, 172
diagnosis x, xi, xii, xvi, 4, 39–45, 54, 70, 71, 75–77, 79–87, 92, 93, 98–100, 103–105, 109–112, 117, 118, 120–130, 146, 150, 151, 182, 183, 185, 191, 203–205, 213, 220
adaptations with diagnosis 150–151, 156–174, 218
with cultural aspects 85
diagnosis and phase 89–100, 206–207
diagnosis, phase, and psychological distance 103–105, 207–210
diagnosis, phase, psychological distance and drama therapy pie 109–110, 210–211
Diagnostic and Statistical Manual of Mental Disorders– 5, *see* DSM–5

Dickinson, Paige xi, xvi, 27, 59, 119
discussion xiv, 7, 19, 23, 32, 37, 49, 53, 66, 70, 81, 90, 107, 109, 110, 111, 118, 119–120, 128, 132, 133, 134, 141, 150, 152, 156, 167, 169, 180, 186, 189, 192, 200, 201, 210, 211, 215, 221, 244
  open ended questions 4, 53, 119–120
  close-ended questions 119–120
  wait-time 169
disorganized thinking 151, 168–169, 218, 230
distance xi, 18, 29–32, 37–38, 58, 61, 65, 67–68, 84, 100–110, 112, 114, 116, 118, 122, 137, 139, 163, 167, 183, 202, 207–212, 215, 220
diversity xi, xvi, 145–174
doubling 68, 178, 233, 235
drama games 15–16, 32, 37, 55, 61, 64, 99, 110, 113, 117, 126, 138, 165, 166, 167, 170, 20, 225–244
drama therapy pie vii, xvi, 21, 33–38, 44, 105–114, 122, 189, 202, 208–213
dramatic play 15–18, 21, 23, 28–29, 48–50, 170
dramatic projection 24, 28–29
dramatic reality vii, 21–24, 28, 38, 61, 124–126, 128, 130–135, 137–140, 165, 167
DSM–5 xvi, 39–42, 44–45, 71, 80–81, 111, 141, 162, 174, 203
Dunning-Kruger effect 64
DvT, *see* developmental transformations

E

elbow-to-elbow 199
embodied life maps 63, 226, 227, 229, 230, 233
embodiment xi, 24, 26–29, 32, 38, 44, 108–109, 115, 116, 156, 210, 211, 213
emotion sculpting 59, 66, 238
emotion spectrogram 59, 237, 238, 239
emotion thermometer 59, 236, 237, 239
emotional spaces 63, 236, 237, 238
emotional orchestra 38, 228, 243
emotional triggers 238
empathy 4, 8, 18, 24, 29–30, 45, 61, 65–68, 71, 119, 127, 130, 133, 134, 149, 235–239
empty chair x, xiii, 64, 225, 228, 229, 233, 236, 244
Emunah, Renee xiii, xv, xvi, 6, 14–20, 35, 59, 62, 63, 136, 138, 140, 201
environmental triggers 163
epilepsy 161–162
ethics xi, xvi, 145, 149, 163, 175–201
ethnodrama 186, 189, 190, 192, 221
evaluation of participant 77, 93, 123–141
executive functioning (EF) xv, 25, 45, 51–65, 81, 111, 183, 201, 221
  metacognition 52–57, 60–65, 81, 112, 113–114, 121, 122, 132, 212, 214
  attention 48, 52–56, 58, 60, 62, 65, 108
  sequencing 52, 57, 63, 64, 65, 114, 166, 169, 234–235
  shifting attention 48, 52, 56, 110, 132, 227–228
  working memory 52, 53–55, 65, 114, 151, 165–166, 218, 235
emotional regulation (ER) xv, 19, 28, 31, 41, 43, 44, 52, 57–59, 60–63, 78, 101–103, 106–107, 134, 169, 183, 207, 209–210, 221, 235–239
  behavioral regulation (BR) xv, 52, 59–61, 63–65, 111–112, 114–122, 180, 183, 197, 201, 212, 221, 223, 225–227
emotional attention set-shifting 62–63
  inhibition 52, 60–61
  initiation 52, 60, 65, 110, 113, 114, 226–227
  self-reflection 26, 52, 61–62, 65, 147
  task planning and organization 52, 63–65, 227

task monitoring 52, 63–64, 65
task examining 64
existential factors 9, 14

F

Family Education Rights and Privacy Act (FERPA 186–188, 196, 221, 222
Fedder's four 57, 166, 169, 227, 229, 230, 232, 233, 239
fine motor functioning 151, 156, 218
first aid 162
flashback 88, 103–104, 163, 198
flexibility 15, 36, 45, 50–51, 76, 78, 133, 135, 149, 225, 229
flow experience 50
follow the leader 166, 228, 240, 241, 243
fortunately/unfortunately 110, 166, 169, 228, 229, 230, 231, 232, 233, 234, 235
four corner dash 38, 226, 240, 241
freeze and justify 61, 110, 226, 229, 231, 233
future projection 104, 232, 234, 239, 244

G

Glennie, Eveline 160
global functioning xii, xvi, 39, 45–71, 76, 78, 81
go 170, 226, 228, 235, 241
go around 51, 115
Goldberg, Elkhonon 52–55
Grainger, Roger 26, 30
gross motor functioning 150, 156, 218
group cohesion 9, 13, 51, 110, 133, 183, 220

H

hand squeeze 111, 120, 166, 234, 240, 241
see also pass the pulse
healing the wounds of history xv
Health Insurance Portability and Accountability Act (HIPAA) 107, 172, 186, 187, 193, 196, 209, 221, 222
hula hoop/bubble walk 200, 240, 241
hula hoop pass 240, 243

I

ICD, *see* International Classification of Disorders
IEP Checklist 160–161, 219
improvisation xiii, 15, 16, 28, 33, 35–38, 44, 46, 48, 50, 58–59, 61–62, 64, 76, 105, 110, 118, 125, 132, 150, 154, 164, 165, 167, 182, 184, 186, 189, 199, 221, 227, 229, 231, 236, 239, 242, 244
integrative five phase model 14–20
phase one: dramatic play 15–17, 35, 37, 44, 88, 93, 95, 97, 98, 99, 100, 102, 103, 105, 106, 110, 111, 113, 117, 118, 121, 128
phase two: scenework 16–17, 99, 100, 102, 138
phase three: role play 17–18, 35, 128, 136, 138
phase four: culminating enactment 18–19, 103
phase five: dramatic ritual 19, 35, 99, 100, 103
International Classification of Disorders xvi, 39–45, 71
imaginary audience 95, 125
imitative behavior 9, 12
imparting information 9, 11–12
installation of hope 9–10, 18
interoception 51
interpreter 146
see also translator
interpersonal learning 9, 12–13

J

Johnson, David Read xiii, xv, 15, 21, 62, 120, 185
Jones, Phil 21, 22, 24–33, 38

K
knots
  see tangling
Klein, Gary x, 47

L
Landy, Robert 153
language comprehension 151, 152–153, 169–170, 218
life-drama connection 17, 24, 32, 37, 48, 107, 109, 112, 120, 128, 137, 138, 140, 141, 167, 186, 210, 211, 212, 221, 233
Linehan, Marsha 61
locus of control (LOC) 43, 46, 68–71, 80, 81, 90, 91, 111, 113, 114, 203, 212, 225, 239

M
machines 38, 44, 166, 231, 232, 234, 240, 241, 243
magic box 116, 227, 232, 234, 237, 238, 243
magic if 16
  see also what if
magic scarf 165, 230
magic screen 38
magic tube 49, 230
mandated participant 179–180
mandated reporter 188, 192, 202
memory
  episodic memory 54
  long term memory 53, 55
  procedural memory 54
  short term memory 27, 54
mirror neuron system 26, 30, 66, 108
mirroring 56, 62, 110, 166, 228, 236, 237, 238, 240, 24, 242, 243
mobility impairment 150, 151, 171, 218
morals 175–176
Moreno, Jacob xiii, 21, 46, 49
multicultural 154
murder 117
museum guard 56, 226, 228, 229, 232, 240, 243
  see also night at the museum

N
NADTA website 183
narradrama xii, 177
narrative transportation 38, 119
night at the museum 56, 226, 228, 229, 240, 242, 243
  see also museum guard
North American Drama Therapy Association (NADTA) code of ethics 145, 163, 175, 178–186, 189–201
Nowicki, Stephen 68–70, 114

O
older adults 27–28, 49, 68–70, 103, 170–171
ordinary reality 22–23, 38, 124–129, 132, 165
overdistance 31, 37, 68, 100, 101, 104, 105, 110, 112, 114, 118, 207, 212

P
pass the pulse 111, 120, 166, 234, 240, 24
  see also hand squeeze
pass the sound/pass the movement 56, 228, 241, 243
pattern ball passing 57, 166, 228, 235, 243
Pendzik, Susana vii, xv, xvi, 16, 21–24, 28, 38, 123–141
people-shelter-storm 166, 226, 228, 231, 235, 243
personification 24, 28–29, 126
Piaget, Jean 15, 170
play xi, 6, 15–16, 21, 23–26, 28–29, 38, 43, 50, 55–58, 61–62, 69, 92, 95, 108, 110, 125, 158, 164, 166, 170, 177–178, 189
play (as in a written play or performance) xiv, xv, 20, 33, 35–38, 62, 79, 106–107, 108, 164, 180, 184, 187, 189, 190, 192, 194,

209–210, 220, 226, 229, 232, 234, 237, 238, 239, 242, 243
playback theatre ix, xv, 18, 32, 35–37, 38, 67, 154, 184, 230, 236, 237, 243
playspace 15, 16, 21, 23
playwriting 57, 182, 184, 190, 220, 232, 239
playing field, even 150
poor clinical judgment 176, 177–178
pop toob conversation 200, 225, 236, 241, 242, 244
Post-Traumatic Stress Disorder 51, 103, 117, 146, 162, 172
power differential 149–150
preoperational stage of development 15, 124
principle of competence 181–185
  competency of knowledge and skills 182
  cultural competence xvi, 28, 199, 145–202, 216
professional development 182
principle of confidentiality 186–193, 221
participant artifacts, storage 186, 192–193, 221
principle of informed consent 193–196
principle of physical contact, role-play, and other drama therapy activities 197–201, 222–223
principle of responsibility and respect 181
projective activities/interventions 37, 186, 221
proprioception 51
psychodrama ix, x, xiii, xiv, 18, 23, 32, 33–34, 37, 38, 46, 68, 100, 114, 117, 119, 153, 177, 180, 184, 229, 230, 236, 237, 239
psychological distance xi, 30, 31–32, 37–38, 100–105, 109–110, 122, 183, 207, 210–211, 220
psychophysical gesture 66
PTSD, *see* post-traumatic stress disorder

R

reading ability 164, 194
reality testing 105, 124–125, 151, 167, 208, 218, 233
replaying scenes 23, 59, 70, 200, 229, 231, 233, 234, 235, 243, 244
resistance 4, 7, 16–17, 19, 87, 117, 125, 198
ritual 6, 19, 24, 99, 115–116, 118, 121, 136, 154, 181, 213, 214
  opening ritual 115
  closing ritual 120
role xii, xv, 6–7, 11, 16, 18, 23, 24, 27, 28, 65, 68, 78, 94, 110, 114, 119, 124–128, 131, 135, 137–140, 149, 153, 169, 171, 185, 195, 214–215, 222, 225, 227, 229, 230, 232, 233, 235, 236, 237, 242, 244
role inventory 65, 153, 227, 229, 232, 233, 234, 235
role model 7, 17
role method ix, xii, 114, 153, 195
role play 6, 11, 15, 18, 24, 28–29, 35, 68, 92, 114, 119–120, 136, 138, 197, 222, 225, 229, 236, 237, 244
role repertoire 16, 18, 65, 114, 127, 132, 133, 134, 214
role reversal xii, 23, 68, 94, 114, 117, 149, 225, 236, 242
rolesort cards 227, 229, 230, 232, 233, 235
role theatre of life 65, 227, 229, 232, 233, 234, 235
Rotter, Julius 68

S

Sawyer, Keith 46–49
scene with three props 227, 229, 232, 235, 243
Scheff, Thomas 30
sculpting 59, 66, 104, 225, 227, 228, 229, 230, 232, 233, 234, 235, 236, 237, 238, 239, 238, 239, 241, 243
  emotion sculpting 59, 66, 228, 236, 237, 238, 239

past-present-future sculpting 104, 232, 234, 235, 239
sculpting a concept 229, 236, 241
sculpting conflict 225, 241
sculpting a continuum 232, 234, 235, 238, 239
sculpting goals 104, 227, 229, 230, 232, 233, 235, 239
self-reflection 52, 61–62, 65, 147
Seligman, Martin 42
sensory integration (SI) 25, 45, 51, 111, 112, 113, 123, 212, 240
sensory motor system 26
service animal 151, 171–174, 218–219
Siegel, Daniel 53
six-key model xvi, 123–141, 195, 214–215
key one: passage 124–125, 130–135, 137–140, 214
key two: quality of dramatic reality 125–126, 131–132, 134, 135, 137–140, 214
key three: roles and characters 126–127, 131–135, 137–140, 214–215
key four: content pattern-plot, themes, conflicts, symbols 127–128, 131–135, 137–141, 215
key five: response 128, 131–135, 137–138, 140, 141, 215
key six: meta-reality 129, 131, 135, 138, 139, 140, 141, 215
six-part story method (6PSM) 165, 230, 231, 232, 233, 234, 235
six-word memoirs 63, 227, 234
social media 45, 93, 175, 181, 186, 191, 193, 221
socializing techniques 9, 11, 12
social-emotional reciprocity 225, 241–244
sociodrama ix, xiii, xiv, xv, 23, 32, 37, 38, 46, 68, 104, 114, 153, 229, 230, 236, 237, 239
soliloquy 38
spectrogram 59, 166, 230, 234, 235, 237, 238, 239
Spolin, Viola xiii
spontaneity xi, xiii, xvii, 15, 24, 36, 45, 46, 49–50, 71, 78, 81, 100, 110, 111, 112, 113, 122, 125, 211
spotlight effect 95, 125, 137
Stanislavski, Constantin 16, 21, 29, 66, 229
strengths-based 39, 42–45, 71, 76, 77, 78, 89–92, 94, 141
storytelling 154, 165, 167, 244
group storytelling 166, 169, 229, 230, 231, 234, 235, 244
supervision 67, 89, 93, 149, 184–185
swoosh-bong 166, 228, 229, 235, 241

T

tactilely defensive 199
tangling 116, 170, 197, 233, 240, 241, 243
theatre games, *see* drama games
therapeutic relationship 3, 4, 9, 10, 36, 93, 96, 97, 103, 116, 147, 148, 205, 216
Title IX 186, 188, 196, 202, 221, 222
to tell the truth 167, 233
touch, use of in interventions 99, 110, 157, 163–164, 175, 179, 196, 197–202, 222, 223
touch as a sense 49, 51, 171, 199
translator 150, 160, 217
see also interpreter
transformation 24, 33, 135
trauma 19, 30, 45, 51, 58, 67, 77, 103, 104, 105, 117, 125, 146, 151, 154, 162–164, 165, 166, 168, 175, 185, 199, 208, 218
treatment planning xi, xvi, 39, 44, 45, 53, 71, 75–94
STOMO 77
traditional treatment planning 76–78
treatment goals 33, 45, 76–77, 92, 96, 97, 111, 195, 205, 206

treatment objectives xvi, 4, 45, 53, 75–79, 87, 92, 93–94, 95, 122, 123, 131, 133, 141, 170, 195, 205
trust falls 99, 170, 241, 243, 244
two truths and a lie 167, 233

U

underdistance 31, 38, 67, 100, 104, 105, 110, 118, 207
universality 9, 10, 81, 136

V

vagus-nerve stimulator (VNS) 161–162
values 175–177
verbal processing 5, 32, 33, 38, 121, 213, 214, 215
visual-impairment 157–158
Volkas, Armand xv
Vygotsky, Lev 15, 28–29, 124, 170

W

warm-up 7, 23, 31–32, 37–38, 51, 56, 92, 101, 102, 104, 109, 110, 113, 115–118, 181, 199, 207, 211, 213
what if? 16, 29
  see also magic if
Weininger, Otto 16, 29
wheelchair 145–146, 156–157, 172
wheelchair ramp 157
who's the leader? 166, 228, 233, 241, 243
willing suspension of disbelief 29
winds are blowing, the 110, 118, 145, 229, 241, 242
wise mind 61, 230, 233, 236, 237, 238, 239, 241

Y

Yalom, Irvin 5–19, 33, 136, 138, 140, 201
Yalom's Eleven Therapeutic Factors 14–Sep
  altruism 9, 10–11
  catharsis 9, 14, 33
  corrective recapitulation of the primary family group 9, 11
  existential factors 9, 14
  group cohesiveness 9, 13
  imitative behavior 9, 12
  imparting information 9, 11–12
  installation of hope 9–10, 18
  interpersonal learning 9, 12–13
  socializing techniques 9, 11, 12
  universality 9, 10, 81, 136
"Yes, and..." 36, 44, 110, 126, 132, 133, 150, 229, 231, 233, 242
yes-no-you 166, 169, 228, 230, 235, 242

Z

zip-zap-zop 56, 104, 166, 169, 228, 230, 235
zone of proximal development 170

www.ingramcontent.com/pod-product-compliance
Ingram Content Group UK Ltd.
Pitfield, Milton Keynes, MK11 3LW, UK
UKHW051334071026
15470UKWH00030B/1803

9 781789 382471